Immunity and Community

Immunity and Community

Identity, Ethics, and Biopolitics

Edited by Bouchra Benlemlih, Mustapha Kharoua,
and Mohamed Belamghari

BLOOMSBURY ACADEMIC
NEW YORK • LONDON • OXFORD • NEW DELHI • SYDNEY

BLOOMSBURY ACADEMIC
Bloomsbury Publishing Inc, 1359 Broadway, 12th Floor, New York, NY 10018, USA
Bloomsbury Publishing Plc, 50 Bedford Square, London, WC1B 3DP, UK
Bloomsbury Publishing Ireland, 29 Earlsfort Terrace, Dublin 2, D02 AY28, Ireland

BLOOMSBURY, BLOOMSBURY ACADEMIC and the Diana logo are
trademarks of Bloomsbury Publishing Plc

First published in the United States of America 2026

A catalog record for this book is available from the Library of Congress.

ISBN: HB: 979-8-216-38044-3
ePDF: 979-8-216-38048-1
eBook: 979-8-216-38045-0

Typeset by Deanta Global Publishing Services, Chennai, India

Contents

Acknowledgments

We owe a profound debt of gratitude to numerous individuals who contributed to this project. First and foremost, we extend our deepest appreciation to the readers and reviewers whose insightful feedback on the chapters enriched this collection. We are particularly grateful to Dr. Rachid Acim, Dr. Mohammed Agzar, Dr. Khadija Belhiah, Dr. Mounir Senhaji, and Dr. Abdelmajid Ridouane for their invaluable suggestions and evaluations of the abstracts submitted to the "ImmUnity & CommUnity" conference, organized in November 2022 by the Research Group on Ethics, Representation, and Politics in Literature and Culture (EREPLIC). As members of the Board of Editors, they not only championed the need for this volume but also dedicated their time to reviewing and editing the conference abstracts. The success of the "ImmUnity & CommUnity" conference was made possible by the generous support of Dr. Mohamed Naji, Dean of the Faculty of Letters and Human Sciences; Dr. Abdelkhaleq Jayid, Dean of the Faculty of Languages, Arts, and Humanities at Ait Melloul Campus; and Dr. Abdelaziz Benddou, President of Ibn Zohr University. We also express our sincere gratitude to the Research Laboratory of Values, Society, and Development (LVSD) Ibn Zohr University, Agadir, Morocco. and its Director, Dr. ELHassan Benabbou, for their unwavering support. Our heartfelt thanks go to all the contributors for their enthusiasm, hard work, and patience throughout the publication process. We are especially indebted to Dr. Sihem Arfaoui, Dr. Boutheina Khaldi, Dr. Laureano Corces, Dr. El habib Louai, Dr. Monir Birouk, and Mourad Maimoune whose thoughtful reviews considerably improved the quality and lucidity of the chapters. A special note of appreciation goes to Dr. Anouar Majid for his illuminating keynote speech at the conference. Professor Majid deserves special thanks and recognition for writing the foreword and for the insightful advice, encouragement and support at various stages of the project. We also reiterate our profound thanks to Dr. Hassan Mekouar for his initial inspiration and enduring commitment to scholarly and community enlightenment. We are honored to reprint *Seven Circles of Self: A Postscript in Verse* in its entirety, originally published in *Decentering Patterns of Otherness: Towards an Asymmetrical Transcendence of Identity in Postcolonial MENA*

(2016), edited by Najib Mokhtari and Aomar Boum. We gratefully acknowledge Dr. Najib Mokhtari for facilitating permissions and coordinating with Prof. Abdelaziz Benjouad, Vice President and Editor-in-Chief of UIR Press, as well as Ms. Najat Loughlim of UIR for her diligent follow-up. Our sincere appreciation extends to Ryan Dradzynski, Acquisitions Editor at Bloomsbury, and the entire team for their proficiency, flexibility, and support throughout the publication process. Finally, we thank our families and friends for their patience and encouragement over the three years it took to bring this project to fruition.

With gratitude, Bouchra Benlemlih,
Mustapha Kharoua, and Mohamed Belamghari

Foreword

Anouar Majid

Making Sense of a Pandemic

The third decade of the twenty-first century was inaugurated with a big bang, a global epidemic that unsettled the world order and ushered in new forms of authoritarianism and unexpected acts of resistance, many spearheaded by anti-establishment physicians or by long-term lawyer activists like Robert F. Kennedy Jr. Using martial law tactics, governments around the world imposed draconian measures including curfews, social distancing, masking, mandatory vaccinations and a myriad other policies designed to protect public health. We were led to believe that merely breathing air can be a mortal threat. Each country had its own exceptions to these protocols, but one couldn't travel without proving recent infection or vaccination.

As the coronavirus spread freely around the world, humans were grounded and restricted to their homes and narrow vicinities. Skeptics of immunity protocols tried to calm public fears by recommending over-the-counter remedies and alternative protocols, including hydroxychloroquine and ivermectin, but they were hunted out of the main networks of communication and the drugs they recommended were locked up or banned altogether, reducing the world population to supplicant consumers for the novel mRNA vaccines of Pfizer and Moderna. (Moroccans relied mostly on traditional Chinese-made vaccines.) Promised to provide immunity, these vaccines failed to prevent new contagion and reinfections, forcing people to remain dependent on a seemingly unending schedule of booster shots.

As a result, Big Pharma, like the superrich, increased their fortunes, while large segments of the middle class (ironically designated as "essential" workers because they are not part of the laptop class) fell into poverty worldwide. Within a year of the pandemic, USB Global Wealth Management reported that the number of billionaires around the world had grown, and that 2,189 of them owned $10.2 trillion of wealth, while between 88 million and 114 million fell into extreme poverty, defined as living on $1.90 a day or less.

Alex Berenson, a former reporter for the *New York Times*, was one of the people who questioned such mandates, publishing a series of pamphlets to question several of these measures. In part three of his series, *Unreported Truths About Covid-19 and Lockdowns* (November 2020), he reminded us that in the beginning of the pandemic, Dr. Anthony Fauci, the director of the National Institute of Allergy and Infectious Diseases, told the CBS news program *60 Minutes*:

> There's no reason to be walking around with a mask. When you're in the middle of an outbreak, wearing a mask might make people feel a little bit better and it might even block a droplet, but it's not providing the perfect protection that people think that it is. And, often, there are unintended consequences—people keep fiddling with the mask and they keep touching their face.

Soon after, the *New England Journal of Medicine* endorsed this view: "We know that wearing a mask outside health care facilities offers little, if any, protection from infection. . . . In many cases, the desire for widespread masking is a reflexive reaction to anxiety over the pandemic." Despite such unambiguous statements, "health experts reversed course and insisted people must wear masks—whether they were feeling sick or well, whether they were in hospitals or stores or even outside."

Those of us who lived in the United States at the time recall that Dr. Fauci had promised that the new mRNA vaccines would prevent transmission, even though the French virologist and Nobel Laureate Luc Montagnier insisted that such vaccines could not stop transmission and that vaccinated people would become asymptomatic carriers intensifying, rather than abbreviating, the pandemic. This meant a financial bonanza for the drug companies selling those vaccines. As reported in Robert K. Kennedy Jr.'s best-selling book, *The Real Anthony Fauci: Bill Gates, Big Pharma, and the Global War on Democracy and Public Health* (2021),

> on October 7, 2021, Dr. Robert Malone, the inventor of the mRNA vaccine, complained in a tweet that America's people were almost utterly blind to the floods of adverse vaccine events that were killing and debilitating their countrymen: "The real problem here is the damn press and the internet giants. The press and these tech players act to manufacture and reinforce 'consensus'

> around selected and approved narratives. And then this is being weaponized to attack dissenters, including highly qualified physicians."

Professor Didier Raoult, the Marseille-based physician and probably the world's most cited expert in the field of infectious diseases, quickly published *Epidémies: vrais dangers et fausses alertes* (March 2020) to remind us that the frantic race to develop a vaccine may very well be a fool's errand since vaccination policies vary among nations and sometimes vaccines turn out to be more dangerous, even lethal, than the threat they are supposed to prevent. Dr. Raoult cites the case of President George W. Bush who was so terrified by the threat of smallpox (because of a film produced by John Hopkins called *Dark Winter*) as a bio-weapon unleashed on the world by the likes of Saddam Hussein that the US military ended up inoculating its members and needlessly killing a hundred of them and causing dangerous heart inflammations in many others.

Writing and publishing furiously as if he were living in truly apocalyptic times, Robert F. Kennedy Jr. followed his book on Dr. Fauci with one titled *The Wuhan Cover-Up: And the Terrifying Bioweapons Arms Race* (2023), building on President Eisenhower's famous warning against the military-industrial complex arguing that "a powerful syndicate, composed of government public health technocrats, a rapacious pharmaceutical industry, military and intelligence officials, and media and social media titans, appropriated awesome new powers to override constitutional and civil rights, censor information, suppress dissent, and engineer compliance with arbitrary diktats." It didn't escape Kennedy that Eisenhower himself was, in some way, echoing C. Wright Mills who had already warned about "a permanent war economy" in his 1956 classic, *The Power Elite*. "For the first time in American history," Mills wrote, "men in authority are talking about an 'emergency' without a foreseeable end." These "crackpot realists," as Mills called these power-hungry men, "have constructed a paranoid reality all their own."

Today, the "biosecurity agenda" that unites "Western public health regulators, military and intelligence agencies" is "the organizing principle of the post–Cold War military-industrial complex—or, more accurately, the military/medical-industrial complex." Is it, therefore, surprising that soon after the election of Donald Trump in 2016, Dr. Fauci gave a speech at Georgetown University, ominously predicting "a surprise [infectious disease] outbreak" during the presidency of Trump?

Dr. Fauci's statement would not be interpreted through dark lenses had there not been a long-standing effort to manufacture novel viruses in order to contain them in what is known as gain-of-function, a practice that is technically not allowed in the United States. But the statistical work of Karina Reiss and Sucharit Bhakdi in *Corona, False Alarm?* (2020) doesn't inspire confidence in the US government's agenda, or even in the West's proclamations for democracy. Not since the Second World War, they argued, were civil rights as severely restricted. The World Health Organization urged people to protect themselves with new gene-based vaccines that had never been tested for human use, or that "truly effective medication hardly exists against any viral disease and that vaccination against seasonal flu is increasingly recognized as being ineffective or even counterproductive." As Dr. Raoult tells us in *Epidémies*, no one knows why flu-like viral infections seem to be seasonal affairs. Infectious diseases, he says, are tied to ecosystems. What complicates matters even more is that human beings, like apes, are made up of billions of viruses and bacteria. To predict outcomes in such a complex environment, as mathematicians try to do with their fashionable modeling, has nothing to do with true scientific thinking.

The authors of *Corona, False Alarm?* were so alarmed by their findings that they concluded with a somber note that captures the sense of helplessness that descended on us during those dark days. "We are bearing witness," they said, "to the downfall and destruction of our heritage, to the end of the age of enlightenment."

Not all is lost, now that Robert Kennedy Jr. has been appointed by President Trump to oversee the US Department of Health and Human Services. Kennedy and his colleagues in charge of critical units such as the CDC, FDA, and others—mostly anti-establishment scientists and physicians during the Covid-19 pandemic—are determined to take on Big Pharma (which has the most powerful lobby in the United States) to protect American citizens and question vaccine narratives and other practices. We also need to use the classic analytical tools of the humanities and social sciences to explain what Reiss and Bhakdi tell us about the apocalyptic ramifications of the Covid-19 world order. This book is an essential contribution to this necessary discussion. With chapters based on papers delivered at an international conference titled "ImmUnity & CommUnity" that took place in Agadir, Morocco in 2022, the book makes significant strides in illuminating the Covid-19 pandemic and what it meant at many levels. The chapters collected in this volume showcase brilliantly why a rigorous study of the humanities and social sciences is indispensable if we want to go beyond the echo chamber of global headlines that disinform more than they enlighten.

Introduction

Bouchra Benlemlih and Mustapha Kharoua

Roberto Esposito, in *Terms of the Political: Community, Immunity, Biopolitics*, notes that "th[e] immunitary *dispositif*, this demand of exemption and protection, which originally concerned the medical and juridical fields, progressively extends to all sectors and languages of our life, until it becomes the coagulating point, both real and symbolic, of contemporary experience" (2012, p. 4). The driving force of this collection is rooted in the close and problematic connection between Immunity or in its Latin formulation, immunitas, which emerges as the contrary, the reverse of communitas. While the two words derive from the term munus that signifies "gift," "office," and "obligation," the tension between immunization processes and the communal or the collective nourishes the need to define immunization in terms larger than the natural reliance on antibodies that fight external viruses or other threats.

The volume consists of chapters based on papers delivered at the international conference titled "ImmUnity & CommUnity" that was organized in November 2022 by the Research Group on Ethics, Representation and Politics in Literature and Culture (EREPLIC) of the Research Laboratory of Values, Society and Development (LVSD) at the Faculty of Letters and Human Sciences, Ibn Zohr University, Agadir/Morocco. It includes contributions that supplement the ongoing debate on the representation of communities' ethics, biopolitics, necropolitics, the emigrant body, the social body, and network society during, and in the aftermath of, the disrupted time of Covid-19, all while intersecting with uneven power relations, globalization, and the modern nation-states. The *complexity* of each of these entities and the interplay among them bring into focus the insufficiencies apparent in the understandings of the concept of "immunity." New directions are then explored within and between each of these disciplines to do justice to the increasingly fluid and interdependent nature of our fast-changing postmodern world. The transformative ideas of immunity highlight its expanding scope, the mode of potentiality and the multitude of ways in which communal identity is being recomposed in a world of complex contagions and the virality of misinformation. The title of the collection defines the major conceptual directions of the volume: "Immunity and Community" emphasizes the connotative interdependence between the notions of "community" and "immunity," while "Identity, Ethics and Biopolitics" offers new configurations of immunity/immunization and opens up new inroads into unexplored fields of critical practice, beyond "echo chambers" and media misinformation.

In scope, the collection explores identity-related dynamics that pertain to immunizing communities worldwide. It draws new cartographies of immunity and community while construing the ramifications of the sanitary conundrum beyond the contours of the medical, thus attesting to the way in which the field of humanities brings further dimensions to bear on the pandemic. Given the ethical and critical prerogative to grapple with the repercussions of the crisis, contributors challenge the medical understanding of "community immunity" or "herd immunity" to excavate further implications from the recesses of history. They confirm that the existence of immunization dates as far back as the Greek era and extends well into the modern times, assuming new meanings across distances of time and space. Alongside historical genealogies and besides the attempts at laying bare the frameworks maintaining the power-relations in existence on both local and global scales, literary representations, philosophical explorations and critical analysis constitute a promising "cure," a good antidote that helps communities come to terms with the aftermath of the pandemic. To that end, the volume reorients critical energies toward their literary and philosophical significance, calling into question the biopolitics of protection that is marred by the unequal distribution of vulnerability in the public sphere. The question of immunity described here centralizes the pervasiveness of immunity as a concept that has triggered long-running debates about the shift from the demands for recognition to the ethico-political intricacies of life preservation. Just as attempts at sustaining life claim to guarantee the individuals' security in order to keep the community safe, they compromise the very sense of relationality they purport to defend when divisions erupt from within.

In so doing, contributors assert that immunity involves contradictions experienced, identified, and confronted by groups and individuals through the many aspects that determine the connotative interdependence between the notions of "community" and "immunity." The complexity of such association locks the two concepts in a critical double bind: they navigate the space between political demands for the right to freedom and basic needs for protective security. Although it has generated persistent calls to stop the relentless cycle of immunization, a process whereby the founding principles of the community are jeopardized, this turbulent in-between has also raised concerns about the pressing need to maintain *naturally* invulnerable collectivities. The rising tension between immunization processes and the communal or the collective thus warrants a redefinition of immunization in terms larger than the natural reliance on antibodies that fight external viruses or other threats. Modern technologies of protection have granted unparalleled attention to the preservation of life, a move that stems from the growing risk of infectious elements that infiltrate not only the individual body, but also other realms including the body politic and the social body. Each system is forced under the power exercised by globalization and the modern nation-states to close off within its protective boundaries. Increased crossovers, social reforms and transformations of everyday practices as well as socio-economic fragility further assert our conviction that immunity entails disrupted identity.

The collection provides creative space at the intersection of medical studies, sociology, philosophy, postcolonial studies, literary studies, critical theory, discourse analysis, and globalization studies, and explores new directions within and between each of these disciplines. The idea of "immunity" is a conceptual lynchpin running through "community" as a very diverse textual constituency, highlighting the process of becoming, the mode of potentiality and the multitude of ways in which "community" is being recomposed during and after Covid-19, a period that has already dictated a great many transformations. The volume thus offers a particularly remarkable variety in the topics it tackles and in the social and cultural contexts it covers. This is to be specifically seen in its two significant characters. First, authors from parts of the world as Morocco, Italy, Slovenia examine issues of "immunity" and "community" and ethical and bio/political representation throughout the period of disruption and its aftermath caused by the Covid19 pandemic. Second, the collection examines the ways in which the concept of immunity persists in such a complex context as the postcolonial condition, the posthuman age and technosociety, or in Heidegger's terms, *Gestell* society, thus maintaining, in the process, a rich conjunctural focus on sociological, philosophical, and critical approaches and the discursive economy of literary texts. As modern technologies of surveillance have taken their toll on Chrononormativities, the innermost details of the everyday, it becomes all the more pressing to redirect critical lens to the procedures of administering all aspects of life.

The texts in this collection, separately and collectively, inscribe immunity and community in an open-ended dialogue. Our contributors construct active literary spaces to bring into play a wide-ranging number of critical perspectives that connect biopolitics, ethics and the shifts that are rupturing to being and subjectivity, particularly as they are experienced on the scale of a global pandemic in the new juncture of a globalized world. The essays variously revisit, update, and reaffirm the literary, sociological, philosophical, and cultural theoretical works of prominent academic intellectuals as Roberto Esposito, Roland Barthes, Martin Heidegger, Manuel Castells, Maurizio Albahari, Bernoux Pihlippe, Abdelwahab El-Messiri, Michel Foucault, Achille Mbembe, Samir Amin, Judith Butler, Walter Benjamin, and Giorgio Agamben. This variety of critical approaches results in insightful readings as they unravel knots and tease out various threads of ethical and bio/political representation of the communal or the collective during, and in the aftermath of, the disruptions resulting from Covid-19. The creative textual forms thus emphasize how sovereign power exerts its extensive control through distancing measures and how particular community members undergo exclusionary inclusion along alterity lines. Topics and issues associated with immunity and community (such as biopolitics, media, the logic of action, globalized network society, *technosociety*, ethics, the immigrant body, social body, global networks of power, autoimmunity, and institutionalized immunization), are treated in ways that serve to remind readers that the subject of immunity has come to embrace a much larger set of intellectual positions than is commonly presumed, and that it can bring into conversation very diverse scholarly agendas and critical practices.

This is an engaging study that focuses on the substantial output of literary texts, media, and cultural practices to celebrate the complexities of the interdependence between "immunity" and "community." It provides creative space within and beyond the larger matrix of the literature on pandemics, putting on display the variety of global immunities and suggesting some of the ways in which various approaches would be fruitful in connecting identity, ethics, and biopolitics with the poetics in the context of post-Covid-19 pandemic.

Chapter 1 in this volume "Techne or Politeia? Some Notes on Roberto Esposito's Hermeneutic of the Pandemic" sketches the idea of a pandemic society. It emphasizes the link among "network," "technology" and "pandemic" as potential basic features of our society. In this chapter, Agostino Cera inquires into the way the network society (Manuel Castells) corresponds to a *technosociety* or *Gestell* society, rather than a mere technological society. By

Gestell society—according to Heidegger's definition of technology as Gestell/Enframing—he means a social-epochal framework within which technology emerges as the "subject of history" Günther Anders). Given its technological imprimatur, a globalized network society turns into a pandemic society: an ideal incubator of pandemic phenomena. The network society emerges as a potential pandemic society precisely insofar as it is *de facto a Gestell* society. If homologation/homogenization is the necessary premise of a safe globalized interconnection, then the shell of the network society could hide the seed of an anesthetized society. The real face of the pandemic society could be that of a unary world (Roland Barthes): the social-epochal framework where "all becomes one." Cera discusses how this framework aims to immunize (Roberto Esposito) itself against the *difference,* because difference emerges as the real virus from which a pandemic society must necessarily defend itself. This unary world looks like Byung-Chul Han's "*transparency society*": an "inferno of the same" where the Other turns into an Alien and finally into an Enemy. Anthropologically speaking, Cera asserts, the pandemic society corresponds to the scenario within which the human type "Bartleby"—someone who can affirm "I would prefer not to"—becomes impossible.

In Chapter 2, "The Sociological Approach to Collective Behavior in the Context of the Coronavirus Pandemic: A Critical Review to the Concept of the Logic of Action in French Sociological Literature," Sidi Mohamed El Hassani reflects critically on how the rapid transformation characteristic of our current era has increased the uncertainty of life, making every rule subject to change and replacement. For El Hassani, the logic of action, as a concept, signifies a shift in the paradigm through which social action has been generally approached. This shift in perspective, which first emerged in the sociological theory of organizations during the second half of the last century, involves rethinking action through the prism of uncertainty and necessitates linking action to the actor, imbuing it with subjectivity and making it open to interpretation according to the specific logic of each situation. Previously, theorists connected action to the general system, which is the bureaucratic organization governed by fixed rules. In such a system, actors found themselves facing predetermined templates and models of action that they were compelled to adhere to in their actions. In the same vein, the author argues, the context of uncertainty in life under the epidemic compels people to react rather than act. Practices such as confinement, mask-wearing, and disinfection, instead of being inherently natural, do not fit into the ordinary register of design; they align more with a framework of differentiation, encompassing not only modes but also the logic of action and encouraging the consideration of situations, anticipation, and adaptation. For Elhassani, our traditional toolbox for reacting and managing events is no longer adequate and needs updating.

The only certainty in all this tumult is that the world has been deeply marked by the mutated corona virus inasmuch as it called upon the very worst in humans. Deciding who lives and who dies, the urge to open the economy at any human cost, the vulnerability of senior community to the pandemic, vaccines' availability to the Global South, human traffic crises on international borders and other hot issues all point to an ethical crisis in the Western paradigm and a retrogression regarding the human donnée therein. In Chapter 3, "The Concept of Man in the West Amid the Pandemic, a Hyper-Phenomenon in Nature or an Epiphenomenon to It?," Moulay Abdessadek Ahlbentaleb explores major ethical and philosophical dilemmas that overwhelmed humanity amid the outbreak of different variants of the new corona virus in its global echoes. Through Egyptian scholar Abdelwahab Elmessiri's criticism of modernist secularist discourse, Ahlbentaleb offers insight into the true worth of Man at paradigmatic moments throughout Western intellectual trajectory. The pandemic raises questions about the value of human existence in the face of a wild anarchic capitalism that does not abide by any theory of value. The endeavor is to test the extent to which the human banners of enlightenment, celebrating a common humanity, have been depleted in favor of a cold and greedy economic order, its unjust social structures, and a new concept of Man alienated from his human essence in times of adversity.

In Chapter 4, "Denied Personhood: The Necropolitical Production of Disposability in Mediterranean Migration," Rachid Benharrousse attempts to theorize the immigrant's body not only in a status of life in death but also in constant autoimmunity. These bodies are perceived as capable of withstanding inhuman conditions until the latter becomes thought of as their normal condition; the containment within overcrowded small spaces, police brutality and harassment, death, imputations, the inexistence of toilets, and the lack of nutrition establishes that the immigrant bodies must be excluded from the civilized space. Hence, community negates the same subjects that ground its continuity. Benharrousse discusses how immigrant body becomes the materialization of the rupture between community and immunity. To confirm this claim, he deploys Esposito's thought to engage contemporary theories of biopolitics toward a novel theorization of the immigrant body.

Mohammad Belamghari and Sara Tabza's coauthored Chapter 5, "Pandemics and Socioeconomic Reforms: A Comparative-Historical Perspective on Infectious Diseases' Impact on Societies," in which they make reference to literary texts and archives as prominent historical documents that play a significant role in shaping affected communities' cultural imagination. The documentation attests to the way in which pandemics have promised to effect change at the social level in key historical moments that far antedate our times. Belamghari and Tabza's study employs a comparative-historical analysis to examine the impact of pandemics such as the Black Death of the Middle Ages, the Spanish Flu of 1918–19 cholera in the nineteenth century, and Covid-19 of the early twenty-first century. The results show that while these outbreaks have spurred positive changes such as advancements in public health systems and the acceleration of digital transformation, they also constitute definite setbacks as they exacerbate existing inequalities and divisions. By unraveling the complex interplay between pandemics and societal dynamics, the study underscores the dual nature of infectious diseases as both destroyers and catalysts for socio-economic reform.

In Chapter 6, "Slovenian Crime Fiction in the Time of the Covid-19 Pandemic and Neoliberalism," Primož Mlačnik brings to the fore the prominent role of fiction. Drawing on Jacques Derrida's and Roberto Esposito's conceptualization of the immunitarian paradigm, Mlačnik untangles the complexities that bring together detective tropes and neoliberal ethos during the Covid-19 sanitary predicament. His reading of Tadej Golob's novel *The Virus (2020)* indicts those who pretend to care for the public good while serving their individual ends. The chapter delineates the kind of unique characterization whose self-serving and self-disciplined acts result in autoimmunization. Under the charge that the infiltration of the ideals of neoliberalism are grounded in a realigned detective/criminal binary, the ensuing alliance between the Slovenian authoritarian state and neoliberalism is condemned for inducing the first wave of the pandemic.

In a world characterized by processes of globalization and mobility beyond all borders of closure, poetry also has a crucial role in redefining the complex association that locks the concepts of "community" and "immunity" in a critical double bind. Conceived as a "postscript in verse" for the collection of critical essays Najib Mokhtari and Aomar Boum edited in 2016 under the title: *Decentering Patterns of Otherness: Towards an Asymmetrical Transcendence of Identity in Postcolonial MENA,* Hassan Mekouar's "Seven Circles of Self: A

Postscript in Verse" presents itself as a meandering reflection on meanings of "self" in relation to the "other," with multiple references ranging from Plato and Dante to Descartes's *cogito ergo sum*, ending with Walt Whitman's "Song of Myself," and borrowing from Moroccan folklore, literature and depth psychology. With its original title now restored, the seven-part poem posits that "self" is a dynamic process that both precedes and includes "community," and that both "community" and "immunity" can only make sense when they are examined through the lens of a "self" that is part of a social, cultural, or biological community.

Immunity and Community: Identity, Ethics and Biopolitics offers fresh insight into identity-related dynamics with regard to immunizing communities worldwide. The themes of the collection highlight that there is a complex and intertwined relationship between immunity and community while putting on display the variety of global immunities and suggesting some of the ways in which various approaches would be fruitful in connecting identity, ethics and biopolitics with the poetics in the context of post-Covid-19 pandemic.

References

Esposito, Roberto. *Terms of the Political: Community, Immunity, Biopolitics.* Translated by Rhiannon Noel Welch. New York: Fordham University Press, 2012.

Mokhtari, Najib and Aomar Boum, eds. *Decentering Patterns of Otherness: Towards an Asymmetrical Transcendence of Identity in Postcolonial MENA.* Rabat: Université Internationale de Rabat, 2016.

1

Techne or Politeia?

Some Notes on Roberto Esposito's Hermeneutic of the Pandemic

Agostino Cera

Premise

This chapter, which is part of a broader work (Cera 2022), focuses on the *hermeneutic of the pandemic*. Its main claim is that an adequate interpretation of the pandemic phenomenon—that is, a *techno-centered* one—gives birth to positive outcomes on the ontological, political, and ethical levels. In other words, acquiring the appropriate perspective to investigate this phenomenon (to establish "from which standpoint should the pandemic be observed/evaluated") will contribute to determining its nature/essence (to understand "what it has been, what it is, the pandemic") and the underlying meaning ("what the pandemic 'meant'").

I will realize this small exercise in pandemic hermeneutic in dialogue with the positions of Roberto Esposito: in my view, one of the few philosophically sound treatments of this topic. Resisting the temptation of real-time interpretation of an ongoing phenomenon (a temptation that risks to result in a sort of philosophical hubris),[1] Esposito was able to get and preserve that minimum "pathos of distance" (Nietzsche 1929, 197–198), that is, that enclave of un-timeliness which is necessary for any philosophical investigation, even when dealing with timely events.

That said, I would like to make it clear that such an appreciation does not mean unconditional agreement. My engagement with Esposito is aimed at presenting an *alternative hermeneutic of the pandemic* to the biopolitically centered—or, better yet, immunologically centered—approach presented in his pages.

"Common Immunity": Esposito's Biopolitical Pandemic

In his 2022 book *Common Immunity: Biopolitics in the Age of the Pandemic* (Esposito 2023), Esposito suggests an interpretation of the pandemic that places it within the "biopolitical paradigm," namely according to that re-actualization of the Foucauldian legacy that he has been advancing for over two decades.[2] On the basis of this assumption, in his view the pandemic has proven to be the forefront of the "contemporary society's propensity to immunize itself," which "has certainly exceeded all imagination, becoming the most significant phenomenon of our time" (Esposito 2023, 4). The pandemic conclusively reveals the interconnection between the legal-political and the medical-biological side, forming "different shades of the same immune syndrome, at once biological, legal, political, and technological" (Esposito 2023, 4).

Among the possible immunity responses to the pandemic challenge—"immunity" understood here in a broad sense, as "*negative protection* of life"[3]—Esposito identifies two: "herd immunity," based on "thanatopolitical principles," and protection through distancing, resulting from a "negative biopolitical choice" (Esposito 2023, 5). Considering both options unworkable without resorting to an autoimmunitarian suppression of the community, he opposes them with an "affirmative biopolitics." This perspective envisions, "for the first time in history," the unique profile of a "*common immunity*," within which "a possible overlap of community and immunity" (Esposito 2023, 14) takes shape.[4] The pandemic generates "a transition that [. . .] is making community and immunity coincide for the first time in history, changing immunity from a blade that cuts through community into its selfsame form" (Esposito 2023, 187).

This brief presentation of Esposito's point serves as a reference point to introduce an alternative hermeneutic: one that revolves around the technology axis, framing the pandemic as a result of the "*Frage nach der Technik*" (Heidegger 1977), understood as an epochal question. More precisely, *our* epochal question. To avoid misunderstandings, it should be clarified that Esposito does not underestimate the importance of technology within the pandemic context, going so far as to argue that "there is a clear relationship between immunization and technicalization, a relationship that is becoming the dominant feature of contemporary political systems" (Esposito 2023, 174). Despite this observation, he believes that such a relationship does not undermine the effectiveness—primacy—of biopolitical-immunological paradigm as a hermeneutic and etiological perspective for deciphering the pandemic phenomenon.

From Utopia to Unavoidability: An Ontology of Pandemic

My thesis is that, despite its merits, the biopolitical-immunological approach is not capable of bringing out the peculiarity of the pandemic as a phenomenon, tending instead to normalize it and thereby diminish its authentic scope and meaning. From a strictly biopolitical perspective, in fact, the pandemic ultimately equates to a reiteration of the inherent dialectic within any political project (or any modern political project, at least), the one existing between the two archetypal modes of managing *bios*, namely *communitas* and *immunitas*, which are semantically inextricably united already from the etymological root in the term *munus*—"with its meanings 'obligation,' 'burden,' and 'duty,' but also 'gift'" (Esposito 2023, 15).[5] The "contradictory copresence" of these two modes corresponds to indiscriminate openness/contagion and definitive closure/protection, respectively. It is an irrepressible dialectic that finds a point of temporary balance in the historical realization of individual political projects and their institutional articulations. In the face of such an archetype, the pandemic may represent a singularity, but only in the sense of a variation on a timeless canon/*Leitmotiv*. This is the final word of a biopolitically/immunologically centered hermeneutic of the pandemic.

On the contrary, my claim is that by centering the interpretation of the pandemic on the question concerning technology—particularly according to its newest manifestation, roughly coinciding with the advent of the so-called Anthropocene[6]—its real peculiarity, that is, its uniqueness, can be fully brought to light. That is to say, that the pandemic scenario embodies a situation in which, for the very first time, the *pan-immunitarian tendency/temptation* that lies at the basis of any political-community project proves to be something concretely achievable and thus something entirely real. The Covid-19 pandemic certified that such a tendency ceases to be an ideal/utopia to which one can approach with the awareness of never realizing it, transforming it into a concrete goal. This metamorphosis of the pan-immunitarian *telos* from the *hyperuranium* of utopias (i.e., unreal possibilities) to the realm of practicable options (i.e., real possibilities) completely changes the terms of the issue.

I previously mentioned some positive outcomes of this techno-centered hermeneutic, starting with the ontological ones. It is now time to delve into the substance. On an *ontological level*, once placed within the framework of the question concerning technology, the pandemic would be qualified as a *phenomenon*, but not as an *event* (the latter understood in the Heideggerian sense, as an *Ereignis*). It would indeed embody a historical *novum* or *unicum*, and thus a discontinuity, yet not comparable to a real "singularity" (in the sense of Kurzweil) or "paradigm shift" (in the sense of Kuhn), but rather to an extraordinary *detonator/trigger* capable of deflagrating—that is, of bringing out completely—some elements already triggered in the fabric of reality but not yet fully visible, entirely perceptible. My suggestion is to consider the pandemic as an epochal *mechanism*, the latter understood in the literal sense of an enactor of processes, an actualizer of potentialities inscribed within the age of technology. According to a famous definition by Goethe, we could define the pandemic phenomenon as an epiphenomenon (i.e., an effect), while technology would correspond to an "*Ur-phänomen*" (i.e., a cause).[7] Or, expressed in Heideggerian terms, only to technology would be attributed the qualification of *Ereignis*, that is, "a way of revealing" (Heidegger 1977, 12), while the pandemic would correspond to the ontic vanguard of it.

The pandemic phenomenon as such—that is, a global and globalized pandemic, as was the case with Covid-19—proved to be something conceivable but considered practically impossible before its actual manifestation. Something *de iure* (theoretically) possible, but *de facto* (practically) impossible and therefore not truly real (*wirklich*), in the sense of not truly achievable or feasible. Regarding this ambiguous ontological status suspended between reality and possibility, the pandemic phenomenon shows a striking analogy with the watershed event of the new century and millennium: Twin Towers attack on September 11, 2001. In that case too, it was something that before occurring was indeed possible (i.e., imaginable and conceivable), but considered outside the horizon of actual reality. Something real as a possibility, but impossible as a reality (*unwirklich*). In both cases, but particularly in the case of the pandemic, the ultimate cause of this ontological metamorphosis—transforming the idea of a global pandemic from a remote possibility into a concrete and tangible reality—is to be found in technology, namely its most recent development. As a result, the adoption of the techno-centered hermeneutical perspective represents one of the few, perhaps the only, viewpoints capable of deciphering what has happened, highlighting its actual meaning and scope.

I am referring first of all to the way the virus "jumped out," namely due to our relentlessly "challenging"—understood in its Heideggerian meaning, that is, as *Heraus-fordern*[8]—toward natural environments (into which we forcefully insert ourselves, displacing its long-time inhabitants, including viruses) and anthropic environments as well (the violence with which centuries-old rural settlements are overnight transformed into "modern cities," even megalopolis).

Consider then the way the virus spread, going around the world comfortably and rapidly (in business class). The same applies to the pandemic management: from prevention and containment strategies (lockdowns, contact tracing, vaccinations) to attempts to establish an "intra-pandemic normality" through what we could describe as *onlife technical tests*: our relationships—professional, recreational, and emotional—at a distance.[9] Each of these stages speaks the language of an age within which technology establishes itself as the only possible *koinè* (common ground), even as the *pharmakon* of our time: both the problem and the solution, the virus and the vaccine at the same time.[10] Having said that, a possible moral of the pandemic story would sound something like this: "against technology (its excesses), more technology is needed."

It bears repeating: a biopolitical-immunological hermeneutic of the pandemic, as argued by Esposito, risks reading it as yet another variation on a timeless canon/*Leitmotiv* (another succumbing to the pan-immunitarian temptation inherent in any political-community project), namely by underestimating the fact that with the Covid-19 pandemic such a temptation has indeed taken place, that for the very first time it has proved to be a real (*wirklich*) scenario because, for the very first time, the contextual conditions were given for it to happen. It happened—maybe it even had to happen—because, for the very first time, it could truly happen. It was *ontologically real as technologically possible.*

As a trigger and enactor of processes, that is, as a mechanism, the pandemic becomes an index of something that, by causing it, transcends it. I refer to the matter of fact that we live in the so-called Anthropocene, the epoch in which the anthropic factor turns into a variable capable of decisively impacting not only human history but also natural history. In the words of Paul Crutzen, the father of the Anthropocene: "humankind has become a global geological force in its own right," that is, "human activities have become so pervasive and profound that they rival the great forces of Nature and are pushing the Earth into planetary *terra incognita* [unknown land]" (Steffen et al. 2007, 614). Our agency—or better, our "technological omni-power"—inscribes itself not only on the surface but in the heart of the Earth system. It etches the "*chair du monde*" (Merleau-Ponty 1968, 248–251) and thus affects even its stratigraphic evolution. By taking this perspective, the advent of the Anthropocene can be seen as the definitive fulfillment of the "*technisches Zeitalter* (age of technology)" described by the "first generation of philosophers of technology" (Achterhuis 2001, 3),[11] that is a framework in which technology proves to be not only the "subject of history" (Anders 2013, 271–279) but also the subject of nature and thus an *integral epochal phenomenon*. As it defines itself, the true face of globalization reveals traits not only of a "technosphere" but an authentic "technocosm",[12] a framework within which technology rises to a totalizing, and potentially totalitarian, dimension. As just mentioned, an integral epochal phenomenon. Having said that, more than "*Anthropo*-cene" (i.e., Age of Humans, Human Era, *Menschenzeit*), it would be fitting to speak of "*Techno*-cene" and as such the strongest candidate to become the *métarécit* of our epoch, the most faithful expression of the current *Zeitgeist*.[13]

Necessitas facit legem: A Politics of Pandemic

From a *political point of view*, a techno-centered hermeneutic of the pandemic phenomenon enables to highlight the emergence of a *techno-political and post-democratic paradigm*. In this case as well, technological possibility becomes an ontological premise. Something is, exists (it cannot but exist) because for the first time its conditions of possibility exist technologically. Its concrete feasibility makes it something inevitable. Again: ontologically real—perhaps even necessary—as technologically possible. At this level, *reality itself*, as such, turns from *Wirklichkeit* into *Machbarkeit* (i.e., makeability, feasibility).

This brand-new political scenario, this unprecedented governmental dispositive found its ideal laboratory in the Chinese government's management of the pandemic. The Chinese model has tried to prove itself in the field as a potentially optimal option— the most performative and efficient—for governing the pandemic phenomenon, while the latter, on its part, was increasingly taking on the role/function of a vanguard for all those fully global(ized) phenomena with which we will more and more have to contend in the future. Thus, while on one hand the pandemic experience aims to represent a "technical test of technocosm" (Cera 2022), on the other hand techno-political post-democracy—the *techno-Leviathan*—aims to establish itself as the best practice for governing the whole globalization. This is the message inscribed in the Chinese management of the pandemic.

Assuming that the essential goal in managing this phenomenon was to save lives, namely to preserve *zoè* (bare life) even at the expense of *bios* (form of life), the Chinese zoopolitical model[14] presents itself as more efficient because it is unburdened by all the constraints imposed on the Western democratic-biopolitical model. Foremost among them, the protection of human rights and individual freedoms (i.e., *bios*) even in an emergency context where *zoè* is threatened (during a pandemic), that is, the impossibility of suspending or completely bypassing them in the name of the higher "right to health" and/or "to life." The pandemic situation strongly emphasizes the Hobbesian assumption at the basis of the "biopolitical turn," an assumption which "made the preservation of life the epicenter of the political" (Esposito 2023, 85–86),[15] that is established the indisputable primacy of *conatus sese conservandi*. The zoopolitics of techno-Leviathan fully agrees with this assumption, moving from the principle that the reasons of *bios* have no voice—and thus can be, must be silenced—when *zoè* is at stake. Because *zoè* embodies the inescapable condition of possibility for *bios*. As a result, in this particular case not only does "*necessitas non habet legem*" hold, but *necessitas facit legem* or, as Esposito himself recalls, quoting a 1909 essay by jurist Santi Romano, "necessity can be said to be the first and original source of all that is law, such that the other sources are to be considered somewhat derivative by comparison" (Romano 1990, 362—quoted in Esposito 2023, 171).

All these arguments one could be countered by stating that in the long run the Chinese model proved—fortunately—its managerial inefficiency, referring to the implosion of the lockdown system (these quasi-massive lagers), which schizophrenically goes from an inviolable "everyone inside" to a sudden "everyone free." My claim is that things might be different, and the Chinese failure tells another story, proving further and paradoxically instructive insofar as it does not invalidate the zoopolitical paradigm, as it might seem at first glance, but unwittingly confirms it. With its actions, indeed, the Chinese government has shown that it is not yet up to the paradigm it aims to represent to the eyes of the entire world. The logic of *total rationalization*—the only ideology practicable by a coherent techno-politics—has been contaminated, and ultimately hindered, by the presence of axiological residues, by an uncleaned-up set of values not yet purified. The functioning of the Chinese techno-political megamachine has been obstructed by the persistence of an inconsistent (i.e., irrational, or better, unrationalized) factor, that is a value-related antiquarianism such as nationalism. While the Chinese government has shown inflexibility and perfect consistency in organizing lockdowns (which have been applied repeatedly and indiscriminately—literally "without looking anyone in the face"), it has refused to make use of the best (i.e., most rational, i.e. most efficient) possible prophylaxis: that offered by Western vaccines, simply because they are Western. Willingness not to admit Western technological superiority by buying and using its pharmaceutical products, this not yet disposed (unpurified and metabolized) axiological residue was an element of inconsistency and weakness in relation to the model that the Chinese government claimed to implement and propagate. A speck of dust (axiological) that jammed the gear of the megamachine.

If China had been completely consistent with its own *modus operandi*; if it had followed exclusively a rationalized logic, then through the combination of indiscriminate lockdowns and adequate mass vaccination it would likely have achieved total success from a health perspective, leaving, however, huge ethical-political questions on the ground. Even more significant than those already substantial ones raised by the inconsistent and incomplete application of its own model. Paradoxically, the best way to establish its own superiority and thus celebrate its nationalism on a global scale would have been to set aside the traditional principles of nationalism. *A techno-political (globalized) nationalism can assert itself only by denying itself*, suppressing its traditional version.

China's failure to manage the pandemic suggests that fully rationalized handling of global phenomena (i.e., techno-political and post-democratic) does not tolerate the presence of the axiological factor. Such a factor proves to be literally unsustainable within this kind of governance dispositive which, as a consequence, requires *axiological neutralization/sterilization*. In its complete manifestation—that globalized and techno-cosmic of a "normalized state of exception"—the neoliberal model appears to embody one of the features attributed to it by Carl Schmitt a century ago: the age of accomplished globalization risks being truly "the Age of Neutralizations and Depoliticizations" (Schmitt 2007).[16] It cannot be otherwise, under the penalty of renouncing its global and planetary dimension. The management of the cosmomachine cannot tolerate that kind of presence, as axiology in itself eventually proves fatally refractory to the "performance principle" (in the sense of Marcuse), not entirely adaptable to the logic of rationalization.

The pandemic phenomenon according to its Chinese version shows how fully rationalized (i.e., completely decontaminated axiologically) post-democratic techno-politics is poised to become the first concrete example of "cosmotechnics," understanding this as the most suitable dispositive to govern an emerging technocosm.[17]

Technology as a Destiny: An Ethics of Pandemic

The Chinese management of the pandemic thus reveals the growing refractoriness, up to intolerance, of the global "network society"[18] toward the axiological dimension. *Axiological anesthesia* appears to be the swiftest, not to say the obligatory, path to the implementation of a global logic, while a biodiversity of values is something unsustainable for such a system, a luxury it cannot afford, risking its own collapse, its implosion.

At the beginning, reference was made to an *ethical outcome* arising from the adoption of a techno-centered hermeneutics of the pandemic. Concluding these pages, I will delve into that reference. The traumatic clash between the reasons of *zoè* and those of *bios* during the pandemic parenthesis speaks, once again, the language of technology, namely of its newest, exponential development. Willingly or unwillingly, here and now we find ourselves placed (thrown) into an unprecedented condition of technological omni-power, which allows us for an equally unprecedented "planetary management": the transformation of our *oikos*/vital space into an entirely controllable, manageable environment. Into a "standing-reserve."[19] Incidentally, this planetary management—the new utopia decreed by the most audacious front of post-environmentalism ecologism, the so-called Ecomodernism—exactly corresponds to the "autoimmunitarian democracy" spoken of by Esposito (Esposito 2023, 49–82).[20]

It follows that before us unfolds an entirely new ethical scenario, well expressed by *Gabor's law* which was established more than half a century ago by Jacques Ellul and Günther Anders. This law, which both considered the categorical imperative of the age of technology, sounds: "What can be made, must be made. What must be made is inevitable" (Anders 2013, 17). *The technologically possible turns into the inescapable*, that is not only into a reality but into a necessity.[21] Here, and this is the point, emerges another key argument in favor of a techno-centered hermeneutics of the pandemic phenomenon. The threshold marking the beginning of the "*terra incognita*" evoked by Crutzen to explain the birth of the Anthropocene could be expressed by the following question: "Assuming that we are *capable* of doing something, do we also have the *right* or even the *duty* to do it?" Within the Anthropocene/Technocene—the framework in which technology becomes an integral epochal phenomenon, that is, the subject of both history and nature—are we still able to escape this equation? Or are we *de facto* already in a condition where it is no longer a matter of right or duty but of *obligation* (unavoidability) to do what we are able to do? To not be longer able to abstain from doing it? Has the possibility already turned into an obligation? More precisely, has the *technologically possible* (i.e., makeable, feasible) already become the *ontologically necessary* and, above all, the *ethically normative*? Has technology really become our *destiny*?[22]

If that were really the case, our *action*—that is, our capability to act understood as a distinctly human prerogative, a founding feature of the *conditio humana* itself[23]—would turn into mere *execution*: the implementation of options and procedures so rational (rationalized) that they become unquestionable and ultimately inescapable/unavoidable. While we, as executors of inescapable/unavoidable directives (i.e., as perfect "rational agents"), would become bearers of a *new innocence* and a clear conscience: the innocence/conscience of those who can afford to be totally irresponsible because they are totally *not* responsible, or better, because they are totally deresponsibilized (unaccountable). We would all become experts or rather "specialists," in the sense in which Adolf Eichmann pretended to be.[24]

Well, it bears repeating, the novelty of the pandemic phenomenon—the peculiarity of the context in which the Covid-19 pandemic occurred—equates to the fact that, for the very first time, such a scenario ceases to be the subject of speculation and mental experiments to turn into a real possibility and therefore a concrete problem. The (con)fusion between traditionally separate and separable realms—that is: *können* (being able), *dürfen* (having the right), *sollen* (having the duty), and *müssen* (having the obligation)—which takes place with the occurrence of this phenomenon is something that impacts and will increasingly impact the daily life of each of us. Technological omni-power, with its accompanying *ethical omni-responsibility* (who can do everything, is also responsible for everything), is and will increasingly be our normal condition.[25] It is a matter of understanding, and possibly deciding, whether it should become our normative condition as well.

So far, this small exercise in pandemic hermeneutics, whose ultimate purpose—alongside exposing the reasons for a perspective that, in my opinion, is more effective than the biopolitical-immunological one in interpreting the pandemic phenomenon—was to reaffirm the fact that, despite all caution, skepticism, snobbery, the pandemic has demonstrated in the field to be "*fragwürdig*": something that not only is worthy, but probably necessary, to philosophically question.

Assuming, however, that philosophy continues to imagine and want itself as the effort to "comprehend its own time in thoughts" (Hegel 1991, 21), namely that "questioning" continues to be "the piety of thought" (Heidegger 1977, 35).

Notes

1 The case, by now a classic, in this regard is that of Giorgio Agamben: "the Coronavirus philosopher." See (Agamben 2021). We choose to quote the original expanded second edition of his pandemic pamphlet (in Italian), because the English translation refers to the first Italian edition, published in 2020. For a critical discussion of Agamben's positions, see (Cera 2022, 154–178) and, in English (Cera 2023a).

2 Here we refer to the *pars costruens* of Esposito's work, established with the first act of the now famous trilogy: *Communitas, Immunitas, Bios*, namely (Esposito 2019—original edition 1998). For an interpretation of Esposito's work, see (Viriasova and Calcagno 2018).

3 "When we define immunity as a *negative protection* of life, we mean that immunity does not protect life directly—in an immediate, frontal fashion—but by subjecting it to a constraint that diminishes its vital potency, channeling that power within certain borders" (Esposito 2023, 20).

4 Esposito positively distinguishes this common immunity from the "co-immunity" he attributes to Derrida and Sloterdijk, that is the last two stages of those "philosophies of immunity," dealt with in the fourth chapter of the book (see Esposito 2023, 119–156).

5 "Community and immunity are two sides of a single semantic block, which acquires meaning precisely from their tension" (Esposito 2023, 15).

6 For an overview of the main genealogical hypotheses on the Anthropocene, see (Cera 2023b, 54–60).

7 Goethe calls some phenomena "*Urphänomen*" (archetypal phenomena) because "nothing higher manifests itself in the world" (Goethe 1983, 195).

8 "the revealing that rules in modern technology is a challenging (*Herausfordern*), which puts to nature the unreasonable demand to supply energy that can be extracted and stored as such" (Heidegger 1977, 14). From this point of view, little would change if it were to be found that the virus has an artificial origin, that it has "escaped" from a Chinese biomedical laboratory. That possibility, even more sinister, would further confirm the importance of the technology factor, that is, the techno-centered character of this phenomenon.

9 As is known, the term "onlife" (a crasis between "online" and "life") represents one of the key concepts in the philosophy of the infosphere, or the so-called fourth revolution, proposed by Luciano Floridi. Among his many works, you can see (Floridi 2014).

10 As is known, the pharmacological status of technology is the focus of Bernard Stiegler's philosophical work.

11 The reference is to authors such as Heidegger, Anders, Arendt, Ellul, Gehlen, Jonas, Mumford.

12 For the idea of "technosphere," see (Haff 2014). For the idea of "*technocosme,*" or "*règne technique,*" see (Hottois 1984).

13 For the redefinition of the Anthropocene as Technocene, see (Cera 2023b, 61–72).

14 I make use of "zoopolitical" in a literal sense, meaning a political paradigm centered on the category of *zoe*, to the detriment of *bios*. Therefore, not in the positive sense attributed by Derrida (as an antispeciesist politics for all living beings), nor in the negative sense (as a critique of biopolitics) by François Warin.

15 Esposito refers to this Hobbesian assumption, quoting the just-mentioned critique by Warin (taken up by Jean-Luc Nancy), toward the biopolitical paradigm. According to this critique, Foucault "abandons historicity to the point of making biopolitics a metaphysics of life" (Esposito 2023, 93).

16 Esposito also sees technocracy as a vanguard in the current process of depoliticization (Esposito 2023, 172–176).

17 My interpretation of the term "cosmotechnics" is quite different from the optimistic one provided by Yuk Hui and based on an intercultural philosophy of technology hypothesis, inspired by the work of Stiegler. On the topic, see (Hui 2016).

18 According to the Spanish sociologist Manuel Castells, the "network society" represents the standard morphology of our societies and consists of "the social structure that results from the interaction between social organization, social change, and a technological paradigm constituted around digital information and communication technologies" (Castells 2004, xvii).

19 According to Heidegger, "standing-reserve" (*Bestand*) is the interpretation of entities which results from the "challenging" (*Herausfordern*) approach typical to modern technology (see Heidegger 1977, 14).

20 On Ecomodernism, which is headed by the *Breakthrough Institute* of Oakland, California (https://thebreakthrough.org/), see the *ecomodernist manifesto*. Animated by an explicit *technolatry*, the manifesto advocates for geoengineering solutions to ecological problems (Asafou-Adjaye et al. 2015).

21 For Ellul's formulation of Gabor's law, see (Ellul 1980, 207).

22 On this topic see (Jonas 2003).

23 Here I am opting for a strong interpretation of "action," inspired by the work of Hannah Arendt in *The Human Condition* (see Arendt 1958, 175–247). According to Arendt, *zoon politikon* (the human being in its fullness) is different from the *animal laborans* precisely as long as it is able to act, that is, to make an authentic action. Her description and critique of *animal laborans* involves an *ante litteram* warning against the current anthropological perversions of "rational agent," "human resource," "human capital."

24 About Eichmann as a tragically emblematic example of "the pure executor"—one who is capable of carrying out any action in a completely irresponsible manner, using the blunt innocence of their professional duty as both a moral and legal alibi—see (Arendt 2006). *The Specialist* is the title of the documentary on Eichmann realized in 1999 by Eyal Sivan assembling original materials from the Jerusalem trial (Svan 1999). Finally, in the emergence of "the expert" within the pandemic context, Esposito identifies a vanguard of populism in its technocratic version (see Esposito 2023, 13).

25 On the *Ethical Paradox of Omni-responsibility*, understood as an inevitable consequence of the technological omni-power, see (Cera 2023b, 157–162).

References

Achterhuis, Hans (ed.). 2001. *American Philosophy of Technology: The Empirical Turn.* Trans. R. P. Crease. Bloomington/Minneapolis: Indiana University Press.

Agamben, Giorgio. 2021. *A che punto siamo? L'epidemia come politica (nuova edizione accresciuta).* Macerata: Quodlibet.

Anders, Günther. 2013. *Die Antiquiertheit des Menschen 2. Über die Zerstörung des Lebens im Zeitalter der dritten industriellen Revolution.* München: Beck.

Arendt, Hannah. 1958. *The Human Condition.* Chicago: The University of Chicago Press.

Arendt, Hannah. 2006 [1963]. *Eichmann in Jerusalem: A Report on the Banality of Evil.* London: Penguin.

Asafou-Adjaye, John, Linus Blomqvist, et al. 2015. *An Ecomodernist Manifesto.* April. http://www.ecomodernism.org/manifesto-english (accessed January 4, 2024).

Castells, Manuel (ed.). 2004. *The Network Society: A Cross-cultural Perspective.* Cheltenham/Northampton: Edward Elgar.

Cera, Agostino. 2022. *Nella società pandemica. Prove tecniche di tecnocosmo.* Fano: Aras.

Cera, Agostino. 2023a. "The Pandemic Society, or the Difference as Taboo." In P. A. e Castro (ed.), *The Social World after Covid-19*, 10–27. Newcastle: Cambridge Scholars Publishing.

Cera, Agostino. 2023b. *A Philosophical Journey into the Anthropocene: Discovering Terra Incognita.* Lanham/Boulder/New York/London: Lexington Books.

Ellul, Jacques. 1980. "The Ethics of Nonpower." In M. Kranzberg (ed.), *Ethics in an Age of Pervasive Technology*, 204–212. Boulder: Westview Press.

Esposito, Roberto. 2019 [1998]. *Communitas: The Origin and Destiny of Community*, Trans. T. C. Campbell. Stanford: Stanford University Press.

Esposito, Roberto. 2023 [2022]. *Common Immunity: Biopolitics in the Age of the Pandemic.* Trans. Z. Hanafi. Cambridge: Polity Press.

Floridi, Luciano. 2014. *The Fourth Revolution: How the Infosphere is Reshaping Human Reality*. Oxford: Oxford University Press.

Goethe, Johann Wolfgang von. 1983. "Theory of Color." In D. E. Miller (trans.), *Scientific Studies (Goehte Collected Works vol. 12)*, 157–298. New York: Suhrkamp.

Haff, Peter K. 2014. "Technology as a Geological Phenomenon: Implications for Human Well-being." *Geological Society Special Publications* 395 (1): 301–309. https://doi.org/10.1144/SP395.4.

Hegel, Georg Wilhelm Friedrich. 1991. *Elements of the Philosophy of Right*. Trans. H. Barr Nisbet. Cambridge and New York: Cambridge University Press.

Heidegger, Martin. 1977 [1954]. "The Question Concerning Technology." In W. Lovitt (trans.), *The Question Concerning Technology and Other Essays*. Trans. W. Lovitt, 3–35. New York and London: Garland Publishing.

Hottois, Gilbert. 1984. *Le signe et la technique. La philosophie a l'épreuve de la technique*. Paris: Aubier.

Hui, Yuk, 2016. *The Question Concerning Technology in China: An Essay in Cosmotechnics*. London: Urbanomic.

Jonas, Hans. 2003 [1979]. "Toward a Philosophy of Technology." In R. C. Scharff and V. Dusek (eds.), *Philosophy of Technology. The Technological Condition: An Anthology*, 191–204. Oxford: Blackwell.

Merleau-Ponty, Maurice. 1968 [1964]. *The Visible and the Invisible. Followed by Working Notes*. Trans. A. Lingis. Evanston: Northwestern University Press.

Nietzsche, Friedrich Wilhelm. 1929 [1886]. *Beyond Good and Evil*. Trans. H. Zimmern. New York: The Modern Library.

Romano. Santi. 1990 [1909]. "Sui decreti-legge e lo stato di assedio in occasione del terremoto di Messina e di Reggio Calabria." In *Scritti minori volume primo: diritto costituzionale*, a cura di G. Zanobini, 349–377. Milano: Giuffrè.

Schmitt, Carl. 2007 [1929]. "The Age of Neutralizations and Depoliticizations." In G. Schwab (trans.), *The Concept of the Political (Expanded Edition)*, 80–96. Chicago: The University of Chicago Press.

Sivan, Eyal. 1999. *The Specialist: Portrait of a Modern Criminal* [documentary].

Steffen, Will, et al. 2007. "The Anthropocene: Are Humans Now Overwhelming the Great Forces of Nature?" *Ambio* 36 (8): 614–621. https://doi.org/10.1579/0044-7447(2007)36[614:TAAHNO]2.0.CO;2.

Viriasova, Inna and Antonio Calcagno (eds). 2018. *Roberto Esposito: Biopolitics and Philosophy*. New York: SUNY.

2

The Sociological Approach to Collective Behavior in the Context of the Coronavirus Pandemic

A Critical Review to the Concept of the Logic of Action in French Sociological Literature

Sidi Mohamed Elhassani

Risk constitutes a fundamental aspect of human existence; however, its prevalence and complexity have intensified in tandem with the technological advancements characterizing contemporary society. Accidents, technological and environmental disasters, crime, terrorism, and epidemics are examples of these risks. We must not forget about risks in our daily lives: we wonder who we will marry, what we will study, what career we will pursue, how we will be financially secure in retirement, and even what we should eat or drink. Our desire to minimize risk shapes our thoughts and behaviors. We need to be protected and "prevention is better than cure"; out of this obsession, behavioral styles and ways of behaving emerge, brought about by an increasingly differentiated environment in response to alienated living conditions or different cultural interpretations of these conditions.

When analyzing road users' behavior, for example, linking their actions to formal regulations—such as the Highway Code—permits a clear distinction between normative behavior and violations. In contrast, in high-risk contexts such as epidemics, behavior is less a matter of rule reproduction and more a response to emerging, unfamiliar conditions. In such cases, individuals do not simply adhere to pre-existing norms; rather, they develop what may be termed a *logic of preventive action*—a behavioral orientation grounded in anticipatory reasoning and strategic adaptation. This shift entails adopting new modes of thinking and enacting behaviors that may contradict previous norms—such as avoiding handshakes as a gesture of greeting. Here, behavioral evaluation is no longer benchmarked against conformity to social norms, but rather against the potential to mitigate risk. The normativity of an action thus becomes determined by its capacity to prevent harm, rather than by its resemblance to socially codified expectations.

This reframing is tied to the broader sociological understanding of *risk*—defined as the possibility that the future may be altered or disrupted, either by human intervention or by natural forces. While individuals may not always exercise control over such events, they can at least adopt measures to anticipate or minimize their consequences. Historically, human beings have evolved as intuitively social actors, relying on a framework of norms, rituals, and rules in relatively stable and sedentary environments, where the margin of risk was limited. These relatively secure conditions enabled the repetition of shared practices, the reinforcement of normative sanctions, and the valorization of piety, often at the expense of critical reflection.

This normative "toolbox"—composed of inherited concepts, rules, and rituals—has allowed individuals to make social judgments and navigate their everyday realities. However, in crisis contexts such as pandemics, individuals are confronted with the realization that this inherited repertoire is insufficient, if not entirely obsolete. In response, they are compelled to shift toward a more personalized, reflective logic—developing individualized strategies to confront uncertainty and adapt to rapidly evolving conditions. This epistemological rupture extends beyond the individual and implicates the broader social structure itself.

Accordingly, interpreting behavior through the lens of *risk* involves a specific epistemological stance: it is not only about examining how society perceives and responds to risk, but also about how sociologists construct explanatory models of action under conditions of uncertainty. This requires a reconceptualization of behavior as an expression of situated rationality, embedded in a logic of action attuned to emergent threats.

Discussions surrounding social behavior in pandemic contexts must thus also be understood as discourses on the constitution of a logic of action informed by social distance. This logic is composed of values and rituals, behavioral patterns, emotional registers, lifestyles, and embedded power relations. It is widely recognized that theoretical frameworks—whether scientific or lay—function as tools for making sense of the world. They are not only descriptive but also orientational: they guide action, define what is relevant or irrelevant and distinguish between real and false problems. This holds true for lay actors, social scientists, and institutional bodies alike.

Nevertheless, sociological analysis of action is frequently confronted with a core epistemological dilemma. On the one hand, it is tasked with analyzing systems of interpersonal interaction along a synchronic axis—one that identifies and differentiates actions based on a fixed initial state of the system under investigation. On the other hand, it must simultaneously account for the diachronic axis—acknowledging that social interaction is dynamic, that actors evolve through engagement, and that the system itself is subject to continual transformation. As Menger (2014, 15) notes, this temporal dimension of action raises fundamental questions not only about the identity of the actors but also about the evolving nature of the interactional situations that bind them.

Before such questions can be addressed theoretically, the underlying problem must be clearly situated within its conceptual framework—namely, that of *uncertainty* and its correlates, as experienced in a horizon of unpredictability. This framework is animated by what might be called the paradox of sociality in uncertain conditions. Given that sociality is predicated on proximity, the imposition of physical distancing disrupts the very conditions under which social relations are typically formed and sustained.

This gives rise to critical questions: How is sociality to be understood when physical proximity and intimacy are curtailed? To what extent can the *logic of action* be seen as a meaningful manifestation of agency within a context defined by uncertainty? What are the theoretical underpinnings of this concept in the sociological tradition? On what grounds can we justify its application to pandemic conditions? And, from an epistemological standpoint, how valid is the concept as a lens for analyzing phenomena such as social distancing?

These questions do not merely invite abstract theorization; they demand a fundamental reconsideration of the frameworks through which we interpret action and interaction in uncertain times.

Theoretical and Paradigmatic Foundations of the Sociology of Action

The concept of *logic of action* occupies a prominent place in the social sciences, where it is frequently employed to denote the underlying principles, rationales, and justifications that inform and guide human behavior. These justifications are neither fixed nor universal; rather, they reflect a plurality of rationalities in the Weberian sense, shaped by varying socio-cultural and historical contexts. Although the origins of the concept are long-standing, it was not fully elaborated into a coherent theoretical framework until its formal development within the sociology of organizations—most notably through the work of Philippe Bernoux in collaboration with Henri Amblard and Gilles Herreros, culminating in their 1996 publication *Les nouvelles approches sociologiques des organisations* (Amblard et al. 2005).

This theoretical contribution sought to overcome the enduring dichotomy between actor and system—a structural legacy of the broader individual/society or part/whole dualism that historically divided sociological thought. Early sociological paradigms tended to polarize along these lines: the individualist tradition, which begins with the actor to explain social phenomena, and the collectivist approach, which takes society as the starting point of analysis. The theory of action logics presents an alternative perspective by emphasizing the situated and interpretive nature of action, thereby moving beyond reductive binary frameworks.

Before engaging with the specifics of this theory and its implications for understanding action in organizational contexts, it is essential to first clarify the etymology and intellectual genealogy of the concept of *logic of action*.

The Context of the Emergence of the Concept

The term *logic* has philosophical roots that trace back to Aristotle, who, in his work *Organon*, defined it as the science of valid inference—deducing new truths from established premises. This foundational definition resonates with contemporary understandings of the *logic of action*, which generally refers to the internal rationale or meaning embedded within human behavior. Every action, even those that may appear senseless or irrational, possesses a latent logic discernible through engagement with the actor's subjectivity—a process Max Weber conceptualized as *verstehen* (interpretive understanding).

Anthropologist François Laplantine similarly asserts that anthropology, in its investigation of human behavior, seeks to uncover the implicit rules underlying action—rules not immediately observable but accessible through abstraction and conceptualization (Laplantine 1993, 147). This move from concrete to abstract transforms everyday behavior into a domain of theoretical inquiry. As such, anthropological logic diverges from common sense by constructing rational discourse that seeks patterns beneath surface phenomena.

In the realm of economics, Vilfredo Pareto introduced a distinction between logical and non-logical actions in the early twentieth century, a contribution later echoed in organizational theory (Amblard et al. 2005, 199). Similarly, Mancur Olson developed a framework for understanding *collective action*, illustrating how small, cohesive groups can effectively advance their interests in ways that larger, more diffuse groups cannot—particularly within lobbying contexts (Olson 1978). Lucien Karpik contributed by conceptualizing the logic of action as a sequence of means and ends, shaped by diverse rationalities. He emphasized how various organizational goals—economic or otherwise—gain coherence and meaning through this sequential logic (Karpik 1972, 82–105).

From this conceptual framework, the logic of action serves several key theoretical functions:

1. Comparing and evaluating organizational objectives.
2. Relating internal goals to external constraints imposed by socioeconomic systems.
3. Establishing a coherent relationship between an organization and its members, grounded in shared principles of action.
4. Linking individual and collective aims, thereby enabling assessment of both economic outcomes and broader social purposes.
5. Interpreting organizational behavior through reference points such as society, profession, enterprise, and individual actors, and articulating its ideological orientation—for example, rigidity vs. flexibility, realism vs. utopia, or negotiation vs. conflict.

Michel Lallement extends this logic to industrial relations, identifying contrasting action logics in employer associations and labor unions—each grounded in differing interests and purposes. While employers pursue profit maximization, unions typically seek improved living and working conditions. Lallement characterizes this divergence as a duality of action logics within corporate systems (Lallement 2008, 62). Guy Bajoit further refines this typology by distinguishing between:

- The *logic of exchange*, in which individuals or groups negotiate relationships with others holding different objectives, competencies, or resources—

producing cooperation, competition, or conflict depending on the nature of engagement.
- The *logic of solidarity*, whereby actors with shared goals align to strengthen their collective influence, often through functional or contractual bonds (Bajoit 2009, 131).

In sociology more broadly, the intellectual lineage of the *logic of action* can be traced to foundational figures of the late nineteenth and early twentieth centuries. Max Weber, although not using the term explicitly, laid the groundwork by classifying social action according to four types of rationality: instrumental, value-rational, traditional, and affective (Terrier 2009). These typologies reflect a broader individualistic orientation that views society as the emergent product of free and rational agents. This perspective informed the work of Gabriel Tarde, whose *La logique sociale* (1895) expanded on his theory of imitation, and Raymond Boudon, who argued in *La logique du social* (1979) that social phenomena result from the convergence of purposeful individual actions and the often-unintended consequences produced within a social environment.

Despite these varied uses, the concept remained diffuse and lacked systematic theoretical elaboration—except within organizational sociology. This subfield experienced a paradigmatic evolution that gave rise to three key demands:

1. Enriching and moving beyond the classical theoretical corpus of organizational sociology.
2. Addressing the inescapable dialectic of conflict and cooperation within organizations.
3. Developing a synthetic and integrative theoretical framework.

Against this backdrop, the term *logic of action* gained traction in organizational theory, appearing in influential titles such as Philippe d'Iribarne's *La logique de l'honneur* (1989) and Gérard Pavy's *La logique de l'informel* (2002), as well as in the work of Sainsaulieu, Boltanski, Thévenot, Reynaud, and Crozier. This context provided fertile ground for the emergence of what Bernoux and Herreros called the *sociology of the logic of action* in the mid-1990s (Bernoux and Herreros 1993), marking a decisive step toward formalizing the concept as a central theoretical lens.

Two main reasons justified the development of this theoretical project:

1. The imperative of theoretical pluralism—linking, integrating, and bridging concepts, schools, and paradigms rather than isolating them.

2. The need to consider the historical and cultural embeddedness of actors, beyond purely rational or strategic frameworks.

Epistemologically, however, the field of organizational sociology has often been marked by a tendency toward insularity. Bernoux and colleagues critique this dynamic, noting that theorists frequently treat their models as "impregnable fortresses" rather than open systems receptive to dialogue (Amblard et al. 2005, 189). For instance, Crozier's theory of strategic actors, Sainsaulieu's analysis of workplace identity, Reynaud's rules of the game, and Boltanski's consensus theories often remain siloed. Even when citations occur, they are typically superficial and do not permit meaningful exchange.

This intellectual insularity stems in part from the dominance of singular starting points—power for Crozier, regulation for Reynaud, identity for Sainsaulieu, consensus for Boltanski, and networks for Callon and Latour—each becoming almost doctrinal. Yet organizations, like all social phenomena, are multidimensional and thus resist explanation through any single theoretical lens.

Neglecting this complexity results in two major problems:

- Theoretical limitations: Fragmented frameworks hinder a comprehensive understanding of organizations, undermining the credibility and relevance of organizational sociology.
- Practical limitations: A lack of integrative models prevents the discipline from offering actionable insights for practitioners, thereby reducing its perceived utility in managerial and policy contexts.

Thus, the *logic of action* emerges not only as a conceptual bridge across fragmented traditions but also as a necessary response to the evolving complexity of organizational and social life.

A New Epistemological Perspective

Epistemological inquiry, whether grounded in Bachelardian rupture, Popperian falsifiability, or Kuhnian paradigm shifts, has traditionally upheld the principle of scientific coherence as foundational to the legitimacy of scientific knowledge. Theories within this tradition are evaluated based on their internal consistency and their capacity to transcend prior conceptual frameworks. Gaston Bachelard's notion of *epistemological rupture*, Karl Popper's *criterion of falsifiability*, and Thomas Kuhn's *paradigm shift* converge on a common epistemic characteristic: the necessity of transcending existing models. This view entails a rejection of cumulative knowledge-building and a resistance to theoretical reconciliation, particularly by disciplinary gatekeepers who enforce conceptual boundaries.

However, this classical epistemological tradition faced significant disruption in the 1970s with the emergence of so-called *irrational paradigms* (Vaillancourt 2006, 2–4). These paradigms broke decisively from Cartesian rationalism, which emphasized calculation, control, and predictability, and instead inaugurated a more reactive epistemology oriented toward improvisation, innovation, and contextual responsiveness. Prominent contributors to this intellectual shift include Paul Feyerabend, Raymond Boudon, Michel Callon, Bruno Latour, and others who challenged the dominance of rationalist and methodologically rigid frameworks.

Feyerabend, in particular, introduced the radical concept of *epistemological anarchism*, advocating for the validity of all theoretical perspectives—including contradictory ones—as tools for understanding reality (Feyerabend 1979). His provocative declaration "Farewell to Reason" (1987) served as a manifesto for the epistemic pluralism encapsulated in the maxim "anything goes." Similarly, the work of R. Parhe and Michel Dogan championed the transposition of concepts across disciplinary boundaries, reinforcing the same pluralistic epistemological stance.

In this context, Callon (1986) and Latour (1996) developed an alternative approach that linked the epistemic status of scientific phenomena to the robustness of the networks that sustain them. Their *actor-network theory* conceptualizes networks as dynamic relational structures that both reflect and constitute the interactions between organizations and their environments. This perspective redefines collective action as an emergent property of complex socio-technical assemblages.

The emphasis on relationality also characterizes the contributions of Mark Granovetter, who, within the domain of economic sociology, sought to demonstrate the extent to which economic behavior is embedded within social networks. Drawing from Karl Polanyi's concept of *embeddedness* (Polanyi 1983), Granovetter argued that economic exchanges—whether in markets or enterprises—are not autonomous but are deeply enmeshed in interperso[illegible] relationships (Granovetter 2000, 77). He introduced the theory of *the stren[illegible] of weak ties*, emphasizing that the frequency, emotional intensity, and trust characterizing relationships play a pivotal role in coordinating behavior, even within modern, highly structured societies.

From the standpoint of these alternative epistemologies, the integration of diverse theoretical frameworks—such as strategic analysis, consensus theory, and network theory—is not only permissible but desirable. Such integration does not necessitate ideological congruence; rather, it reflects the complex, multifaceted nature of social reality and the analytical need for theoretical pluralism.

In this pluralistic vein, Sainsaulieu introduced the notion of *logique de l'acteur* (actor's logic), referring to the identity-based logics adopted by groups within organizations as they assert their interests, often in adversarial relationships with other groups. In this framework, action is conceived as an expression of pre-existing identities, with logic anchored in the actor's prior characteristics.

However, this static conception is challenged by Amblard and his collaborators, who reject the premise that the actor precedes action. Instead, they adopt an existentialist stance: the actor is constituted through action, not prior to it—*existence precedes essence*. Accordingly, the logic of action is dynamic, evolving alongside the actor's engagement with their context.

> From this standpoint, the theory of the *sociology of the logic of action* posits that organizations cannot be adequately understood through singular paradigms that privilege either cooperation or conflict. Rather, a dialectical approach is required—one that acknowledges the interplay of both dimensions in shaping organizational life.

This theoretical framework reconceptualizes collective action within organizations by integrating both conflictual and cooperative logics. It draws in part on Jürgen Habermas's *theory of communicative action*, developed in response to the question: how is social order constituted? Habermas contends that social systems are not solely products of strategic interest calculations but are also rooted in processes of mutual understanding and cooperative negotiation. Social coordination, in his view, may emerge through influence or consensus, thereby necessitating a plurality of theoretical tools to grasp its complexity.

In sum, the *logic of action* offers a renewed epistemological and theoretical lens for analyzing organizational and social phenomena—one that is attuned to multiplicity, contingency, and the generative power of action itself.

Components of the Logic of Action

A further contribution of this framework is its challenge to the notion of a singular, optimal pathway in processes such as entrepreneurship. Rather than positing a universal formula for success, it recognizes the diversity of trajectories through which enterprises are established. This diversity emerges from the unique configurations of actors and action situations, with each case shaped by specific contexts and goals. As Philippe Bernoux notes, the plural form *logics of action* is intended to highlight this variability and to make conceptual room for the contingencies inherent in entrepreneurial practice.

Moreover, the *logic of action* framework supports interdisciplinary analysis. Its conceptual flexibility enables it to accommodate insights from economics, sociology, geography, management studies, and psychology. Such interdisciplinary engagement is not merely advantageous but essential for a comprehensive understanding of entrepreneurial behavior and the broader dynamics of organizational life.

In sum, the concept of the *logic of action* offers a robust theoretical lens through which to interpret the events and transformations that punctuate organizational life. Whether in response to strategic shocks, failed contracts, or product misalignments, the logic of action provides a means of attributing meaning to events. For instance, the misalignment between a CEO's individualistic logic and a team's collective ethos, an austerity-driven approach to staffing, or a traditional consumer logic out of step with a novel product design—all can be understood as expressions of distinct logics of action (Durand, 2013, p. 124). In this way, the framework not only enhances interpretive capacity but also contributes to a deeper understanding of organizational behavior in context.

Theoretical Extensions of the Concept of the Logic of Action in General Sociology

As previously noted, the concept of *logic of action* has gained significant traction within contemporary sociological discourse. Although it is invoked in diverse contexts and carries multiple connotations, it consistently refers to a theoretical framework that seeks to transcend two traditional and reductionist paradigms of social action: the deterministic structuralist model and the rationalist utilitarian model.

The first paradigm interprets social action—such as patterns of consumption, educational pathways, or occupational trajectories—primarily through the lens of objective structural determinants, including gender, social class, ethnicity, and other ascribed statuses. Within this framework, the autonomy of the actor is largely negated, and the sociologist's role is to reveal the external forces that condition both the formation of intentions and the execution of actions. Agency, in this context, is either marginalized or wholly subsumed under the weight of social structure.

In contrast, the second paradigm emphasizes the rational agency of the actor. It posits that social actions are the result of deliberate, intentional choices made by individuals who possess the cognitive capacity to evaluate alternative means in light of desired ends. Here, the actor is conceived as a purposive agent, exercising free will and making decisions based on cost-benefit analyses that aim to maximize utility. From this perspective, social behavior—whether voting, selecting an educational specialization, purchasing a consumer good, or deciding to have children—is explained primarily through the logic of instrumental rationality.

The concept of the *logic of action*, as developed in more recent sociological work, proposes an alternative to this binary by suggesting a relational and dynamic synthesis. Rather than positioning structure and agency as mutually exclusive, it emphasizes the co-construction of action through the interplay between actors' intentions and the situational, historical, and institutional contexts in which these actions unfold. In doing so, it enables a more nuanced and comprehensive understanding of social behavior, one that neither reduces action to mechanical reproduction of social structures nor idealizes actors as sovereign decision-makers operating in a vacuum.

From the Logic of the Actor to the Logic of Action

Michel Lallement identifies three major trajectories that sociological research on social action—particularly in the French context—has pursued (Lallement 2000, pp. 255–262).

1. The organizational sociology approach

The first trajectory emerges from the sociology of organizations, particularly through the work of Philippe Bernoux, who argues that contemporary sociology has shifted away from a sole focus on the individual actor in organizational analysis, instead privileging the notion of the *logic of the actor*. This concept integrates collective dimensions and identity-related dynamics. Renaud Sainsaulieu, in his influential work *L'identité au travail* (1977), attributes the formation of professional identities to the adoption of shared logics of action by actor-groups (e.g., workers, technicians) within the workplace. According to Sainsaulieu, the alignment of interests, behavioral norms, and values within these groups facilitates the emergence of identifiable social patterns that, during the 1970s, were foundational to workplace culture.

Sainsaulieu's focus on identity formation within organizations aligns with his broader interest in corporate culture, which he conceptualizes through several key assumptions (Sainsaulieu 1997):

- The existence of a shared culture among organizational members;
- The potential for cultural conflict during organizational mergers;
- The linkage between organizational culture and its overarching project;
- The institutionalization process through which organizational culture becomes internalized.

Corporate culture, in this view, comprises a constellation of symbols, representations, values, and interpretive frameworks that guide individual behavior. Far from being externally imposed via human resource strategies, culture is generated through the interaction of individuals with technical work processes and organizational structures. It is thus a collective construct shaped by continual exchanges across various organizational strata (Sainsaulieu 1977, p. 447).

While Sainsaulieu advanced strategic analysis by integrating subjective experience—particularly identity and belonging—Michel Lallement critiques his methodology for privileging the actor while neglecting the situational dimensions of action. From Lallement's perspective, the logic of action is better conceptualized as an emergent property of the relationship between the actor and the action situation. As he notes, "the logic of action varies with situations and is not determined solely by the actors themselves" (Sainsaulieu 1977, p. 447).

In this framework, the logic of action results from the interaction between an actor—shaped by social history and identity—and a situation defined by institutions, norms, and power relations. Bernoux illustrates this with a case study from a workshop at the Berliet company, which included three worker categories: those of agricultural origin, those from working-class backgrounds, and Tunisian immigrants with rural roots. Agricultural-origin workers demonstrated deference to hierarchy, while those from working-class backgrounds were more inclined to contest authority. Tunisian workers oscillated between these two behavioral models, influenced by cultural, familial, and strategic factors. Some shifted their allegiance from an agricultural identity to a working-class one (1982), a transition shaped not only by individual agency but also by broader historical and structural transformations. This example underscores the need to connect micro-level behavior with macro-level social dynamics.

2. François Dubet's sociology of experience

The second research trajectory is exemplified in François Dubet's theoretical contributions, particularly *La sociologie de l'expérience* (1994) and *À l'école* (1996). Building on Alain Touraine's framework, Dubet proposes three interrelated logics of action:

- The logic of integration, which refers to group-based affiliation and the reproduction of collective identities within a given social structure (e.g., students forming identity-based groups within a school).
- The logic of strategy, rooted in market rationality, where actors pursue self-interested goals and develop utilitarian strategies to navigate competitive environments.
- The logic of subjectivity, linked to cultural values and personal commitments to abstract ideals such as citizenship, authenticity, and discipline.

Dubet asserts that these three logics are never entirely isolated but interweave within the actor's lived experience. He refers to this interplay as *social experience*, defined as "the articulation of different logics of action by the actor, resulting in a dynamic that structures their subjectivity and reflexivity" (Dubet 1994). Social action, therefore, resists reduction to any single logic. In a world where no centralizing institution (e.g., the state, the market, or culture) singularly determines behavior, individuals are constantly negotiating between conflicting rationalities.

For example, in analyzing the role of teachers, Dubet notes a shift from role-based identity (derived from institutional expectations) to professional identity (based on personal engagement). Teachers now distinguish between the expectations tied to their formal role and their lived experience of teaching. This creates a duality between two distinct logics of action, further emphasizing the actor's ongoing negotiation between structure and subjectivity.

3. The economy of justifications

The third trajectory is represented by Luc Boltanski and Laurent Thévenot's *De la justification* (1991), which inaugurated the "Économie des grandeurs" (Economies of Worth) research program. Their framework focuses on the normative justifications actors employ during disputes, emphasizing the pluralism of moral and cognitive capacities. Unlike deterministic or purely utilitarian models, their approach assumes that actors possess the reflexive capacity to justify their behavior using shared cultural repertoires.

These justifications are particularly evident in moments of conflict—such as workplace disagreements, political debates, or interpersonal disputes—where individuals invoke general principles to legitimize their actions. Boltanski and Thévenot identify six "orders of worth (1999)," each grounded in a distinct value system, such as:

- The *world of fame*, where recognition by others defines value;
- The *domestic world*, grounded in hierarchical trust and familial loyalty;
- The *market world*, where worth is defined by ownership and competition.

Each of these orders provides a *logic of action*, guiding actors' behavior and shaping their justifications in context-specific ways. Analyzing these justifications thus becomes a way to uncover the hidden normative frameworks that structure everyday social life. In conclusion, sociologists who engage with the *logic of action* paradigm seek to avoid both structural determinism, which assumes the primacy of social systems in shaping behavior, and methodological individualism, which overemphasizes rational calculation. Despite the analytical complexities it entails, this paradigm opens up two important avenues for the study of social action.

First, it facilitates the integration of rationality with identity. Rational action cannot be fully understood without accounting for the actor's social identity, which includes self-perception and interactions with others (Lallement 2000, p. 260). This necessitates an approach that bridges biographical narratives, subjective projects, and intersubjective relations.

Second, the logic of action paradigm contributes to debates on social justice by affirming a pluralistic understanding of rationality. It aligns with John Elster's notion of *local justice*, which argues for context-sensitive criteria in domains such as healthcare or welfare distribution. Elster's example of organ transplant prioritization—based on urgency, potential outcome, or social utility—illustrates how different logics of action can generate competing yet legitimate frameworks of fairness (Elster 1992; Lallement 2000, p. 201).

In sum, adopting the logic of action as a conceptual framework enables a multidimensional understanding of organizational and social phenomena. While originally developed by Bernoux and Herreros (1993) in the context of organizational analysis, and later adapted to entrepreneurial studies by A. Fayolle (2003), the concept serves as a robust starting point for systemic and interdisciplinary analysis.

To investigate the logic of action is to explore the foundational rationalities underpinning actors' decisions. Crucially, the logic of action is not a fixed or deterministic structure. Actors do not exist in isolation from the situations they inhabit; rather, they are constituted through their actions within specific contexts. As such, the logic of action evolves with the unfolding of actions rather than being rooted solely in individual dispositions. This framework thus affirms the coexistence of strategic and cooperative rationalities, emerging from the interplay between two essential components:

- The actor, understood in their historical, social, and cultural embeddedness;
- The action situation, understood as a complex configuration of norms, institutions, and power relations.

From the intersection of these elements, diverse patterns of action emerge, reinforcing the necessity of theoretical pluralism. In existential terms reminiscent of Sartre, the actor does not precede the situation; rather, they are shaped through it. The diversity of situations therefore produces a multiplicity of action logics, justifying a pluralistic and context-sensitive sociological approach.

To What Extent Can Social Distancing Be Considered a Logic of Action?

Drawing upon the study conducted by Mohamed Hilal Al-Hassani and Abdelmalek Ward regarding the impact of quarantine on social interactions in Morocco (Al-Ḥassanī and Ward, 2020), it can be argued that the Covid-19 pandemic significantly influenced the emergence of new logics of action among

Moroccan citizens. The researchers structured their investigation around five principal axes:

Axis I: The Relationship between Individuals' Social Conditions and Their Perception of the Covid-19 Phenomenon

An individual's social context exerts a decisive influence on their perception of events and on the nature of their response to crises that threaten psychological, social, and existential stability. The study's findings suggest that individuals' interpretations of the pandemic are reflexively linked to their daily practices, lifestyle, and socio-economic positioning. Three dominant forms of perception emerged:

1. The pandemic as a normal phenomenon;
2. The pandemic as a sudden and terrifying disruption;
3. The pandemic as a conspiracy, divine punishment, or biological mutation.

These perceptions correspond to distinct social categories. Those perceiving the pandemic as abrupt and alarming were mainly day laborers, students, and informal workers—groups characterized by socio-economic vulnerability. Conversely, those who interpreted the pandemic as routine or ascribed it to conspiracy or metaphysical causes tended to be employed in public or private sectors, professionals, and small traders with more stable livelihoods.

For these latter groups, the pandemic either resembled previous health crises (e.g., SARS, foot-and-mouth disease, mad cow disease) or was understood through metaphysical or political frameworks. This ambivalence reflects a broader cognitive dynamism: a continual reassessment of reality based on religious, scientific, and political references. The multiplicity of interpretations thus illustrates the interplay between social position, available cultural resources, and perceived agency.

Axis II: Responses to the Evolving Dynamics of the Covid-19 Pandemic

This section explores individual responses to the Covid-19 pandemic, which unfolded in two distinct phases. The initial phase was characterized by a perception of the pandemic as a distant threat, leading to various logics of action. Among these were the *logic of dismissal*, which perceived the virus as a geographically confined issue limited to China; the *logic of mockery*, exemplified by sentiments such as "We already struggle with colds—why worry about Covid-19?"; and the *logic of indifference*, which entailed a passive reliance on divine protection and the dismissal of preventive measures. Expressions such as "We ask God to protect and shelter us; we have no power against God's will" illustrate this attitude. These responses reflect a constrained awareness of the global nature of pandemics and demonstrate a lack of comprehension of the interconnectedness of time, space, and risk in the era of globalization.

Drawing on Bajoit's theoretical framework(Bajoit 2009, 131), any logic of action presupposes a degree of agency and a corresponding space for autonomous decision-making. This, in turn, requires a form of detachment from the collective, which can be interpreted as a form of social distancing. However, the concept of freedom within this context warrants further examination. Philosophical and sociological discourses have long debated the distinction between independence and freedom. Many individuals may appear autonomous, yet few truly embody freedom in the deeper sense. Freedom, in this view, entails intelligence—the capacity to apprehend one's environment fully, free from fear, coercion, or the compulsion for security. Strategically, an actor's freedom is proportional to their ability to navigate uncertainty and exert influence over it.

Within the context of a pandemic, viral transmission constitutes a critical domain of uncertainty. Consequently, social distancing may be interpreted not merely as imposed isolation but as a form of liberating action—a strategy to regain control. This challenges the prevailing perception of quarantine as enforced sedentarism and is informed by what Guinchard and Arnaud (2011) term the *domestic paradox*. This paradox emerges from the tension between the private and public spheres—the home and the external world—and becomes especially pronounced during periods of occupational disruption, such as retirement or confinement. Work, as these authors suggest, fulfills multiple psychological functions, most notably anchoring individuals in reality. Its sudden interruption often leads to frustration and existential dislocation.

This perception was most commonly reported among day laborers and informal workers (65 percent), followed by students (24 percent), and public and private sector employees (11 percent). The prevalence of these attitudes among economically vulnerable populations suggests that such logics of action are closely tied to socio-economic precarity. Media representations—particularly unregulated digital content—played a central role in reinforcing the image of the virus as a remote, China-specific phenomenon. Videos associating Covid-19 with Chinese culinary practices, for instance, reinforced the perception of the pandemic as an external, culturally distant event (Al-Ḥassanī and Ward 2020, 261).

> Thus, the pandemic was frequently viewed through the lens of spatial and psychological distance, fostering attitudes of denial, mockery, and indifference. These perceptions underscore the constructed nature of public awareness, heavily mediated by digital platforms and information flows.

A parallel logic—*the logic of supplication*—also emerged, characterized by appeals to divine will and expressions of helplessness in the face of crisis. This response reflects a fatalistic worldview prevalent among both socio-economically disadvantaged and educated segments of the population. Among the respondents, 63 percent of those from stable, educated backgrounds and 36 percent of those from more vulnerable groups, including students and informal workers, reported such attitudes (Al-Ḥassanī and Ward 2020, 261). This worldview tends to foster resignation and submission to misfortunes—be they illness, oppression, or disaster—stemming from a lack of critical understanding and agency.

In the subsequent phase, when individuals began to experience the pandemic "up close," three dominant attitudes were observed:

1. Belief in divine will and predestination some respondents framed the pandemic as a divine test or punishment. One noted: "Human failure to end this pandemic proves it comes from God; it is a punishment for unbelievers and a test of the faithful." Another stated: "Even if a vaccine is found, it is still an act of God's will." Such expressions indicate a limited degree of trust in scientific rationality. These beliefs function as *doxa*—uncritical opinions resistant to epistemological inquiry. In the words of Gaston Bachelard: "Opinion thinks badly; in fact, it does not think. It expresses a need to know and is the first obstacle to overcome in the acquisition of scientific knowledge."
2. Belief in the restorative power of nature Other respondents interpreted the pandemic as a natural corrective. One declared: "It's a natural disaster like a tsunami, and it will lift its burdens from the earth." Another suggested: "It's a natural transformation that transcends human laws." This perspective aligns with environmental determinism and

echoes arguments made by Saifan, who observed that the pandemic accomplished what climate conferences could not: reductions in pollution, the revival of familial life, and a rethinking of the human relationship with nature.

3. Experiences of fear, instability, and insecurity The most widespread response among vulnerable individuals—including day laborers, students, and informal workers—was one of existential insecurity. These respondents felt abandoned by natural, divine, and human actors alike. Their immediate concerns were grounded in their reliance on daily income and direct social interactions for survival. Their sense of injustice stemmed not only from the pandemic itself but from the exacerbation of pre-existing inequalities that it revealed.

Axis III: Individual Perceptions of the Role of Chance in the Covid-19 Phenomenon

This section addresses how individuals interpreted the role of chance and unpredictability in the emergence and consequences of the Covid-19 pandemic. Although most respondents underscored the sudden onset of the pandemic and the unanticipated measures introduced to manage it, their appreciation of the element of surprise varied significantly. Foremost among the unexpected outcomes was the complete cessation of work, cited by 42 percent of respondents. This was followed by the enforced isolation and the disruption of kinship ties, which were emphasized by 22 percent. The rapid global spread of the virus and its severe toll, particularly in developed nations, ranked third at 17 percent. Other less frequently mentioned yet symbolically significant surprises included the closure of schools (6 percent), mosque closures (3 percent), social phobia and fear of others (3 percent), the universality of infection (2 percent), and the uncertainty regarding the pandemic's end (29 percent). Additionally, 39 percent of participants highlighted the generalized sense of panic and societal disarray (Al-Ḥassanī and Ward 2020, 262).

It is unsurprising that work stoppage emerged as the most salient disruption, given its foundational role in ensuring psychological security and social stability. Even those not directly affected by the closures expressed empathy and solidarity with the economically impacted, especially after the shutdown of cafes, factories, and other productive sectors. The discontinuation of kinship visits and the imposition of isolation severely disrupted individuals' capacity to engage in relational and communal life—an essential component of social identity in societies where familial bonds and visitation customs are deeply embedded.

Social distancing, as a policy and practice, became a substantial source of psychological strain due to its effect on interpersonal connection, which serves as a vital source of spiritual and emotional nourishment. According to Clément et al. (2009, 9), the formation of social bonds occurs progressively through three key acts: (1) approaching others and reaffirming ties, (2) initiating encounters and dialogue, and (3) coexisting while maintaining personal integrity. These acts collectively aim to elevate "living together" as the cornerstone of social cohesion.

However, when such processes are disrupted—as in the context of mandated isolation—the entire social model is called into question. Clément et al. (2009, 12) argue that intimacy and solitude are as foundational to human experience as connection and discourse, especially during critical junctures like a pandemic. From a sociological standpoint, social distancing also induces a leveling effect on social hierarchies by neutralizing performative distinctions. In the absence of others, as Sartre famously stated, the private self loses its contrastive definition—"hell is other people" becomes inverted into an existential vacuum. The cessation of social recognition rituals—what Spinoza and later Matheron (1988, 193) identified as manifestations of desire, jealousy, and reciprocity—suspends the dynamics of domination and subordination, fundamentally altering intersubjective relations.

The astonishment at the pandemic's swift global spread and its devastating impact even in highly developed nations reflects the emergence of a new critical awareness. This challenges prevailing assumptions about technological and medical advancement, particularly the illusion that progress necessarily entails resilience to public health threats. The pandemic thus prompts a reevaluation of development paradigms that fail to safeguard against widespread vulnerability.

From an ethical perspective, social distancing confers moral agency upon both healthy and ill individuals, recognizing them as active participants in the collective health landscape. It fosters an ethic of shared responsibility and commitment to the common good (Gross 2017, 1). Within clinical contexts, patients with chronic illnesses have long been seen as co-constructors of their care; during a pandemic, this model extends to the general population. Healthy individuals are encouraged to adopt preventive behaviors not only to protect themselves but also to mitigate transmission risks. This expansion of responsibility constitutes a broad-based therapeutic education, turning each person into a public health actor.

Moreover, individual participation has increasingly extended beyond personal protection to include the evaluation of health policies, volunteerism in clinical research, dissemination of public health information, and critical oversight of governmental responses. In this context, civic education—grounded in values such as citizenship, engagement, and cooperation—becomes essential in countering apathy and fostering collective resilience. According to Albert Hirschman's framework, states are confronted with a binary choice in such crises: either to amplify the *voice* of their citizens or to risk their *exit*, understood as withdrawal and disengagement from public life (Gross 2017, 118).

In conclusion, this analysis underscores that social equilibrium is intrinsically tied to individual stability. Societal cohesion hinges upon the continuity of essential social functions—work, parenthood, civic participation, and both formal and informal networks of solidarity. These elements form the fabric of community life, which must be sustained and adapted even amid profound uncertainty and disruption.

Axis IV: Individual Responses to Quarantine Obligations

Although all respondents identified cleanliness as an essential component of daily religious practice, attitudes toward social distancing and quarantine measures varied significantly across social and geographical contexts. In particular, residents of rural areas exhibited considerable resistance to social distancing protocols, viewing them as disruptive to the core of their relational and moral fabric, which is deeply rooted in emotional proximity and community interaction.

With respect to the concept of quarantine as home confinement, responses revealed clear gendered and socio-economic disparities. Approximately 80 percent of female respondents perceived home quarantine as a normative or acceptable practice. In contrast, 78 percent of male respondents reported difficulty in adapting, citing a perceived infringement on their freedom of movement. Among younger individuals from economically vulnerable backgrounds, nearly 80 percent expressed rejection of the quarantine conditions. Their discontent was primarily linked to structural deficiencies, such as the lack of internet connectivity at home, and economic constraints that made it difficult to satisfy basic personal needs during confinement—such as mobile phone top-up cards and tobacco products.

Despite these challenges, the domestic quarantine period appeared to prompt a form of social and familial reconfiguration. Respondents indicated that fractured or neglected social ties were often restored, as individuals re-engaged with family life and rediscovered forms of marital and parental intimacy. When asked about the most meaningful collective habits developed during this period, 27 percent of participants highlighted the revival or discovery of family cohesion, expressed through shared meals, joint study sessions, communal prayer, and the collective recitation of the Qur'an. Additionally, 15 percent of male respondents noted their increased participation in household labor, reflecting a temporary reorganization of domestic gender roles.

On the level of individual activities, respondents reported a range of newly acquired habits and practices. Foremost among these was independent reading (26 percent), followed by close attention to economic and political developments and updates on the pandemic through television and internet platforms (24 percent). Participation in distance learning and online education accounted for 22 percent. Other activities included religious observance—namely remembrance of God and Qur'anic reading (12 percent)—as well as developing culinary skills among men (10 percent), engaging in physical exercise (3 percent), and increased time spent playing with children (3 percent).

In sum, while home confinement undeniably posed significant challenges—particularly in terms of personal autonomy, privacy, and the severing of ties with extended social networks—it also yielded a set of beneficial outcomes. These include what might be termed "positive rediscoveries," as individuals reconnected with neglected aspects of their inner lives and familial relationships. In many cases, the interruption of external distractions enabled a renewed investment in domestic life and intimate relationships, areas often marginalized by the demands of contemporary professional and social obligations.

Axis V: Individuals' Perceptions of the Present and Aspirations for the Future

Respondents' reflections on the present moment and their projections for the future revealed a division along two primary lines: a moderately optimistic minority and a predominantly pessimistic majority. The optimistic group, comprising 53 percent of participants, grounded their outlook in religious faith, expressing confidence in divine providence and in the potential for society to overcome the current crisis with limited long-term consequences, ultimately returning to a semblance of normalcy.

Conversely, 47 percent of respondents expressed a predominantly pessimistic perspective, shaped by a sense of uncertainty and skepticism regarding the future. This group's outlook is underpinned by their perception of significant structural obstacles to meaningful reform, including entrenched social inequalities and institutional inertia. They cited a lack of political will as a core impediment to change and expressed concern over the nation's ongoing reliance on international financial institutions. Such dependency, they argued, effectively places national resources—and by extension, the country's future—under external control, perpetuating a state of socio-economic vulnerability.

Conclusion

The epidemic, as an extraordinary event with profound implications for humanity at this historical juncture, has disrupted the foundational structures of social life by calling into question prevailing modes of interaction—most of which are grounded in physical proximity and face-to-face engagement. This disruption compels not only a transformation of these interactional patterns and everyday practices but also a reconfiguration of the underlying cognitive and perceptual frameworks that sustain routinized action. Such a shift is essential for cultivating a strategic orientation capable of anticipating future contingencies and managing uncertainty with greater efficacy.

From an academic standpoint, this chapter pursued a dual objective. First, it aimed to present a critical overview of the theory of action logics and its relevance to understanding social phenomena—particularly behaviors emerging under conditions of uncertainty, such as those engendered by a pandemic. We have shown that this theoretical framework enables the transcendence of entrenched dualisms—science/common sense, individual/collective, fact/value, cognitive/emotional, rational/irrational—that often underpin enduring theoretical disputes and obstruct the formulation of integrative perspectives. Notably, it offers an epistemological space where seemingly incompatible interpretations of reality can coexist in a logic of complementarity, rather than mutual exclusion. Second, this work sought to contribute to a rethinking of epistemological paradigms in the construction of theoretical models and conceptual tools. Such models must be attuned to the temporal dimension of human action, with particular attention to its future orientation. Acknowledging the anticipatory nature of action invites a more dynamic and context-sensitive approach to theorizing social life in times of profound uncertainty.

References

Al-Ḥassanī, Mohamed Hilāl and Ward, ʿAbd al-Malik (الحسني محمد هلال، ورد عبد المالك). "Taʾthīr al-ḥajar al-ṣiḥḥī ʿalā al-tafāʿulāt al-ijtimāʿiyya bi-l-Maghrib: Taḥlīl sūsiyūlūjī li-mafāhīm al-ṣudfa wa-l-lāyaqīn" (تأثير الحجر الصحي على التفاعلات الاجتماعية بالمغرب: تحليل سوسيولوجي لمفاهيم الصدفة واللايقين). In *al-Wabāʾ fī al-madīna min manẓūr sūsiyūlūjiyā al-fiʿl* (الوباء في المدينة من منظور سوسيولوجيا الفعل), edited by Idrīs Āyt Lho and Saʿīd Balaʿḍīsh ((225–202 ,(تنسيق إدريس آيت لحو و سعيد بلعضيش. Rabat: al-Maṭbaʿa wa-l-Warāqa al-Waṭaniyya (2020 ,(المطبعة والوراقة الوطنية.

Amblard, Henri, Philippe Bernoux, Gilles Herreros, et Yves F. Livian. *Les nouvelles approches sociologiques des organisations*. Paris: Seuil, 2005.

Bajoit, Guy. *Socio-analyse des raisons d'agir : Étude sur la liberté du sujet et de l'acteur*. Québec: Presses de l'Université Laval, 2009.

Bernoux, Philippe. *Un travail à soi*. Toulouse: Privat, 1982.

Bernoux, Philippe, et Gilles Herreros. "Le changement dans les organisations: entre compromis et pouvoir." *Gestion 2000*, no. 6 (1993).

Boltanski, Luc, et Ève Chiapello. *Le nouvel esprit du capitalisme*. Paris: Gallimard, 1999.

Boudon, Raymond. *La logique du social: Introduction à l'analyse sociologique*. Paris: Hachette, 1979.

Callon, Michel. "Éléments pour une sociologie de la traduction. La domestication des coquilles Saint-Jacques et des marins-pêcheurs dans la baie de Saint-Brieuc." *L'Année sociologique* 36 (1986). http://manuel.boutet.free.fr/innovation2014/Traduction-Saint-Jacques.pdf.

Clément, Michèle, Lucie Géluneau, et Anaïs M. Monica. *Proximités : Lien, accompagnement et soin*. Québec: Presses de l'Université du Québec, 2009.

D'Iribarne, Philippe. *La logique de l'honneur: Gestion des entreprises et traditions nationales*. Paris: Seuil, 1989.

Dubet, François. *Sociologie de l'expérience*. Paris: Seuil, 1994.

Durand, Rodolphe. *La désorganisation du monde*. Lormont: Éditions Le Bord de l'eau, 2013.

Elster, Jon. *Local Justice: How Institutions Allocate Scarce Goods and Necessary Burdens*. Cambridge: Cambridge University Press, 1992.

Fayolle, Alain. *Le métier de créateur d'entreprise*. Paris: Éditions d'Organisation, 2003.

Feyerabend, Paul. *Contre la méthode: Esquisse d'une théorie anarchiste de la connaissance*. Paris: Seuil, 1979.

Granovetter, Mark. *Le marché autrement*. Paris: Desclée de Brouwer, 2000.

Gross, Olivia. *L'engagement des patients au service du système de santé*. Paris: Éditions John Libbey Eurotext, 2017.

Guinchard, Roland, et Gilles Arnaud. *Psychanalyse du lien au travail: Le désir de travail*. Issy-les-Moulineaux: Elsevier Masson, 2011.

Karpik, Lucien. "Les politiques et les logiques d'action de la grande entreprise industrielle." *Science Rationalité et Industrie* (1972). https://doi.org/10.3406/sotra.1972.1860.

Lallement, Michel. "À la recherche des logiques de l'action." In *La sociologie, histoire et idées*, coordonné par Philippe Cabin et Jean-François Dortier. Paris: Éditions Sciences Humaines, 2000.

Lallement, Michel. *Sociologie des relations professionnelles*. Paris: La Découverte, 2008.

Laplantine, François. *L'anthropologie*. Paris: Payot, 1993.

Mancur, Olson. *La logique de l'action collective*. Traduit par Mario Levi. Paris: Presses Universitaires de France, 1978.

Matheron, Alexandre. *Individu et communauté chez Spinoza*. Paris: Éditions de Minuit, 1988.

Menger, Pierre-Michel. *The Economics of Creativity: Art and Achievement under Uncertainty*. Cambridge, MA: Harvard University Press, 2014.

Pavy, Gérard G. *La logique de l'informel*. Paris: Éditions d'Organisation, 2002.

Polanyi, Karl. *La grande transformation*. Traduit de l'américain. Paris: Gallimard, 1983. (1re éd. américaine: 1944)

Prévot, Hélène. "Le mythe moderne au risque de l'anthropologie: bref aperçu des théories de Bruno Latour." *Aspects sociologiques* 4, no. 1–2 (mai 1996). http://www.fss.ulaval.ca/cms_recherche/upload/aspectssociologiques/fichiers/prevot1996.pdf.

Sainsaulieu, Renaud. *L'identité au travail*. Paris: Presses de la Fondation Nationale des Sciences Politiques, 1977.

Sainsaulieu, Renaud. *Sociologie de l'entreprise*. Paris: Presses de la FNSP et Dalloz, 1997.

Terrier, Jean. "Culture et types de l'action sociale." *Revue Européenne des Sciences Sociales*. Consulté le 9 décembre 2009. http://journals.openedition.org/ress/635. https://doi.org/10.4000/ress.635.

Vaillancourt, Raymond. *Le temps de l'incertitude : Du changement personnel au changement organisationnel*. Québec: Presses de l'Université du Québec, 2006.

3

The Concept of Man in the West amid the Pandemic, a Hyper-Phenomenon in Nature or an Epiphenomenon to It?

Moulay Abdessadek Ahlbentaleb

Since its eruption in Wuhan, capital city of the Chinese Hubei province, and its propagation worldwide, SARS-CoV-2 variant triggered urgent concerns within the informed circle of scientific societies and a lot of controversy among both the global public and world policymakers. Notwithstanding the global economic lockdown, the marked social distancing restrictions, and the psychological impact of compulsory confinement, there emerged polemicists with disputable and sometimes indisputable statements, bordering on multiple conspiracy theories. The fact that the virus travels on 5G mobile networks stands no chance against Bill Gates' microchip implantation project as he predicted a pandemic outbreak at the 2015 TED Talk forum. Another polemic is the seepage of the virus from a Chinese virology lab, carried by a going-rogue bat to the infamous Huanan wet market, making it the epicenter of the pandemic worldwide. Some conspiracists went as far as to claim that the virus was originally a biological weapon used by the Chinese against the Americans while, in another version, the Americans imported it to China amid the Military World Games organized in Wuhan in October 2019. Depriving populations of their freedoms, the plotting of big pharma, or world population reduction through pandemics are other conspiratorial schemes that marked the outbreak of the new coronavirus on a global scale.

Embracing such conspiracy theories is rooted in the confused and depressed economic and social conditions of world populations, struck by a deadly unexpected virus whose spectacular spread was difficult to process, let alone to contain. The new social mediatic behavior had its share in propagating infodemics, adding to the unfaith that the global community showed toward equivocal virological experts, alongside dishonest politicians and predatory crisis investors. Yet, aside from the conspiratorial *rationale* underlying the tension amid the spread of the deadly virus, there is some credibility over other issues that the pandemic initiated. Deciding who lives and who dies among the senior community, the urge to relaunch world economy at any human cost, vaccines' inequity and the Global South, and other related issues all point to an ethical crisis in the Western paradigm and a retrogression regarding our common humanity. It is becoming increasingly difficult to ignore how the pursuit of special interests, the cultural transformations of global highly mediatized populations, and the primacy and overvalue all this assigns to sheer private profit-making in hard times could impact human lives on a global scale.

This chapter examines the profound ethical and philosophical challenges that have emerged amid the global spread of different variants of the coronavirus and how the pandemic raises fundamental questions about humanity's true essence within the Western paradigm. Employing a multidisciplinary critical approach, addressing philosophical, historical, social, economic, and scientific dimensions of the pandemic, this chapter navigates the value of human existence, unveiled at paradigmatic secular moments throughout Western intellectual history. Cogitating Western civilizational *malaise* through the lenses of Zygmunt Bauman, Herbert Marcuse, and Abdelwahab Elmessiri in their multiple critical examinations of the ills of modernity and their societal impacts, this chapter modestly contributes to the debate over the degeneracy of the West-led global world order, which has long refrained from promoting an unconditional humanism and a multiculturalism of solidarity in times of adversity. Put differently, it provides a critical reading into Western ideologies and the different conceptions of Man they cultivated, leading to the fatalistic human condition amid paradigmatic secular moments akin to the third millennium's pandemic.[1] This genealogy that discloses the limitations and potentials of what it means to be human would help enlighten the dimensionless fatalities that escorted the pandemic, exclusively in the Global North.

The Secular Paradigmatic Moment in the Wake of the Pandemic

In relation to the idea of progress rooted in the Western context and linked to a specific stage in modern (material) history, Western thought has always struggled in its attempts to provide answers to the final questions facing Man: What is the purpose of existence in this universe? Is it to promote good and prevent evil, as traditional metaphysics suggests? Is it to seek truth and self-knowledge from a Western humanistic viewpoint? Or is it to prioritize unrestrained earthly pleasures like production, consumption, profit, and enjoyment over transcendence? (Elmessiri 2000, 143–144). The Western man's "maturity" from the traditional metaphysics of transcendence to that of immanence (Western modernity) is at the heart of any comprehensive understanding of social change in the West. This is particularly significant since that transition brought about a disoriented existential compass and an utterly disorienting naturalist/materialist worldview that failed to take the human *donnée* into account according to the Enlightenment banners of humanism once dearly upheld. Accordingly, the pursuit of and commitment to the idea of scientific and material progress at all costs took over an outstanding intellectual current within Western civilization that showed an aversion toward history and ideology (Elmessiri 1979, 16). The profound impact of Western civilization is undeniable, leaving a lasting legacy of questioning, innovation, and global influence that has shaped human history. Initially, to be modern

> is to find ourselves in an environment that promises us adventure, power, joy, growth, transformation of ourselves and the world—and, at the same time, that threatens to destroy everything we have, everything we know, everything we are . . . . Modernity can be said to unite all mankind. But it is a paradoxical unity, a unity of disunity, it pours us all into a maelstrom of perpetual disintegration and renewal, of struggle and contradiction, of ambiguity and anguish. (Berman 1983, 15)

The concept of unbridled progress toward a technological utopia raises concerns about a potential imbalance once pro-matter/nature, anti-human, and anti-culture elements were injected in Western critical orientation (Elmessiri 2006: 48). The developments in Western thought since the Enlightenment created an ethical dualism regarding a primal, unconditional Adamic humanity, ultimately proving detrimental even to the natural order it once revered.

Ostensibly, behind every human phenomenon there stands an epistemological model which is an explicit transfiguration of the human conception of the universe. It revolves around three axes: God, Man, and Nature, and stands as the source of unity behind diversity (Elmessiri 2002a, 5). What is reproachable regarding Western modernity is that it bestowed ultimate priority on nature/

matter, subjecting humans to deterministic natural laws (Elmessiri 2002a, 7). Initially, the Western intellectual trajectory started with the magnitude that Mind gained after it replaced God in this cosmological trinity (Elmessiri 1998, 13). Elmessiri qualifies this major shift as a continuous degeneration of modernity away from the early utopian and humanist banners of the early modern age. It moved from the freedom of the human mind, the centrality of Man in the universe, and the belief in his autonomy from nature/matter (1997a, 26) toward bestowing primary importance upon nature/matter, thus subjecting humans to its blind dictates (2002a, 7). All this brings about the birth of the naturalist/materialist Man who is pragmatic, functional, contractual, one-dimensional, tamed, rationalized, reified, and alienated from his human essence (Elmessiri 1997a, 245). As materialism takes hold, society ushers in a new archetype, estranged from his inherent humanity.

For Elmessiri, the Western tendency to deify the human mind in its supremacy over transcendence is a simplistic and reductionist view of the universe, driven by a desire to decompose man back into the fabric of nature, leading to the abolition of the self and ultimately the death of humankind (2002a, 47). Only then,

> [a]ll unique human boundaries collapse, along with human identity and the complex world that contains Self and Other, and wherein human beings exist as responsible creatures who choose between good and evil. A faceless, flat universe with no boundaries emerges, for materialist monism cannot cope with complexities, boundaries, multiple levels and identities, i.e., it cannot cope with what distinguishes human beings as human beings and what sets them apart from all other beings. (Elmessiri 2006, 51–52)

Elmessiri characterizes this Western stance as heralding the end of history after declaring the death of God and the nullification of human autonomy and will (2006, 48). Put differently, it transmutes the human element from a hyper-phenomenon in nature into an epiphenomenon to it, whose existence, although concomitant with, is not causally contributory to the evolution of that hegemonic natural order. In summary of its underlying secular absolutist assumptions affecting the human condition, Elmessiri emphasizes that,

> instead of a metaphysics of transcendence, where the universe achieves coherence and meaning through a centre that is external to it, secularism operates in terms of a metaphysics of immanence, where the centre of the universe is immanent in both humanity and nature or in either. This results . . .

> in an illusory dualism that resolves itself into a monism. Reality projects itself first as an oscillation between a humanity-centred and a nature-centred outlook, between extreme individualism and extreme collectivity, between solipsism and reification, between a self-referential human self that considers itself the locus of immanence and a self-referential physical nature that is considered the locus of immanence. (1996, 44)

To corroborate these secularist tendencies, Elmessiri recognizes that the complex world of shifting dualities such as God-humanity and later on humanity-nature collapses into the organic simple world of monism that is governed by one single principle (1997b, 4). Accordingly, humanity witnessed its downfall according to the different manifestations of the immanentist incarnation of the ultimate divine either in humans or nature. Thus, God's incarnation in one people generated racism while fascism emerged when God incarnates in the leader (Elmessiri 1997b, 7). Elmessiri refers to this Man-centered orientation as solipsistic imperialist monism, "wherein the self-referential human subject deifies itself and declares itself the organizing principle of the world." Later, that self was overcome by what Elmessiri refers to as naturalist materialist monism, wherein the "self-referential natural object arrogates for itself the status of being the only organizing principle," leading to the dissolution of all dualisms (1997b, 6).

Ultimately, the Western mind invented an earthly paradise to deceive the multitudes into deserting transcendence. However, in his zealous industriousness to establish one in which he controls all aspects of his temporality, the materialist, imperialist, self-deifying man ended up living in hell (Elmessiri 1979, 18). Since reality is always richer and more complex than our perception of it, such quest is abortive because it dooms that God-like self to a rapacious materialist exploitation out of greed for wealth and power. In quest of material comfort and happiness, the truth the materialist man seeks becomes rooted in everything that efficiently maximizes production regardless of any human value (Elmessiri 1979, 39). On sacrificing the otherworldly salvation to a material utopianism, accessible here and now, Man becomes a mere commodity as well. Accordingly, different biases in favor of nature/matter against the human factor emerged:

1. Bias toward the material and natural at the expense of the immaterial and human exposes humankind to control, experimentation, and quantification as in the experimental and physical sciences in total disregard of his moral, psychological, or teleological dimensions.

2. A bias that manifests itself in favor of the general, accurate, and universal phenomena to the detriment of uniqueness, diversity, and specificity, because these escape abstraction which is considered necessary for the attainment of general natural laws.
3. Valuing the perceptible, the measurable, and the quantitative, which are amenable to the five senses, calls for the rejection of that which could not be approached with the same degree of scientificity, namely what is complex, qualitative, and indefinite.
4. Looking for simple models, simple interpretations, one decisive cause, a single center of the universe, and reducing phenomena to one variable or principle become the order of the day. This entails the rejection of difference, otherness, and the resulting diversity of paradigms. Thus, centricity around oneness gives way to Bentham's material utility, Adam Smith's profit-making and the accumulation of wealth, Marx's development of tools of production, Freud's *Eros*, Carlyle's heroes, the Nazis' Aryan race, or Zionists' promised land.
5. Bias highly values objectivity, neutrality, passivity, and complete detachment in the treatment of both objects and human phenomena, disregarding moral obligations, passions, human totality, and human inner motives.
6. On the level of terminology, bias manifests itself in a leaning toward a generalized, accurate, descriptive, non-figurative, precise, and unambiguous language in an algebra-like manner (Elmessiri 2006, 33–38).

Demonstrably, juxtaposing isolated events in human history would help disclose the human condition's retrograde position within the Western civilizational context. Accordingly, the Western man's identity was sealed in consistency with those utopian ideals and turned into dystopian realities. The effects run the gamut from the promises of modern life, the dramatic shift from the traditional metaphysics of transcendence to that of immanence, the move from partial to comprehensive secularism, the advent of capitalism, slavery and colonization, indigenous first nations' extermination, aggressive cultural imperialism, two world wars, Western-waged genocides, and postmodernity's evils. The third millennium's pandemic can be regarded as another secular moment in which materialism and progress seem to prevail over being. It prompts introspection into various aspects of human existence, raising thorny questions about human resilience, full adherence to moral principles, and the interdependence of global communities amid *glocal* crises. Philosophically, the pandemic challenges human understanding of individual autonomy versus collective obligation, seeing its huge repercussions on our common humanity. The far-reaching fatalities, recorded during the global combat to contain the pandemic, are dismissive of the myth of an alleged morally driven conduct that characterized the spirit of humanism and the enlightenment philosophy that framed its emergence in the West. Put differently, it raises questions, fears, and concerns in the neoliberal countries about how far all boundaries can be transgressed in devaluing fundamental precepts of human existence in times of adversity.

Ageism and the Italian Scenario: How Capitalism Plagues Public Health

One of the most spectacular manifestations of a universe deserted by God, where defenseless humans were left to fend for themselves, is how the seniors' crisis has been handled in the Western world. It is just unimaginable how defeatist such powerful countries have grown, trying to protect infirm portions of their societies, as international press and media reported. There is no longer room for any amazement, seeing how PM Boris Johnson spread panic among his fellow British citizens, inviting them to bid farewell to their loved ones instead of working to mobilize their close ranks to face the ordeal united (Coleman and Mullin-McCandlish 2021, 183). Understaffed, under-sourced retirement facilities and the corresponding inhuman neglect toward a founding class of the world community solicits some reflection about ageism in a typically materialistic neoliberal first world. Lal *et al.* argue that "COVID-19 has pushed all health systems to their limits, exposing severe gaps in public health infrastructure, even in nations once lauded as the gold standard for readiness" (2021, 61). Prosperous countries in the developed world like Canada, Italy, and Spain demonstrated lack of protocols, total mismanagement, and mishandling resources to lessen the casualties, as the international press revealed.

In *The Psychology of Aging*, Janet Belsky claims that "today we may be living in one of the most-age-friendly ages of all" (1999, 7). The outbreak of Covid-19 just proved the contrary. Statistics from Italy, for example, reveal the dimensions of the infection and the worrying death toll among senior population in alarming figures. Thus said, "of the patients who died, 42.2% were aged 80–89 years, 32.4% were aged 70–79 years, 8.4% were aged 60–69 years, and 2.8% were aged 50–59 years (those aged > 90 years made up 14.1%). The male to female ratio is 80% to 20% with an older median age for women (83.4 years for women vs 79.9 years for men)" (Remuzzi and Remuzzi 2020, 1255). In Highly Covid-19-stricken Italy, the Lombardy province, one of Europe's wealthiest regions, left its health workers unprotected and suffered poor coordinating emergency measures to contain the pandemic amid the overflow of infected patients into hospitals and in retirement homes (Lal *et al.*, 2021, 62–63).

Historically, there was a lucrative side to the blooming of nursing houses in the first world. Those facilities moved from being non-profit, public long-term care institutions, issuing out of the old system of almshouses, into a source of revenue for the new entrepreneurs in the sector of services. Ogden and Adams see that retrogression from an economic perspective whereby, after being a social good, nursing homes turned into a consumable good. Demonstrably, the proliferation of those institutions fundamentally "altered the form and ethos of nursing homes from small, 'mom-and-pop' residences and voluntary facilities, and it changed the politics of long-term care as the new purveyors began to influence finance and regulation policy" (Ogden and Adams 2009, 146). Seeing that the provided services were disastrous, the 2020 pandemic led the graying population toward (un)voluntary large-scale death tolls. It was expected for an originally charitable and humanitarian social practice to fall in the grip of market ethics, where the most vulnerable are turned into assets that could be bought and sold or just disposed of. In this regard, Herbert Marcuse does not see freedom of enterprise, which is an originally fundamental right, as a blessing. Consequently, he continues, as "the liberty to work or to starve, it spelled toil, insecurity, and fear for the vast majority of the population" (1964, 4). Thus, instead of sustaining human dignity, it ended up opening critical social sectors to the ups and downs of the market.

The blind trust in and compliance with the market forces in operation on every level of social service proved impactful on health sustainability and livability. Zygmunt Bauman observes that social inequality intensified along the dissolution of the welfare state, once advocated through Rousseauian *contract social*. He wonders why in the first world prosperity is in concert with all types of social evils, including low life expectancy despite the high quality of life that Western societies promised their multitudes. Drawing parallels between East and West, Bauman notes that,

> in the most unequal societies on the planet, like the United States or Britain, the incidence of mental illness is three times higher than at the bottom of the

> inequality league; they also rank high in their prison populations, the bane of obesity, teenage pregnancies and . . . in death rates for all social classes, including the richest strata. Whereas the general level of health is as a rule higher in wealthier countries, among countries of equal wealth death rates fall when the degree of social equality goes up . . . A truly striking finding is that the rising levels of specifically health-related expenditure has had almost no impact on average life expectancy—but a rising level of inequality does have such an impact, and a strongly negative one. (2011, 38)

Bauman attributes these upheavals to the materialist dictates reigning over the lives of those subject to the state's multiple power apparatuses. Minority groups like the graying population and the associated age-related problems akin to insufficient medical assistance during the pandemic was a recurrent paradigmatic moment that revealed the darkest side of those blind market forces in play.

Exploring the striking differences between the third world and Western societies regarding perception of the elderly is revealing as well. It is startling to see how "permissive" Americans, for example, are when they abandon their parents in the homes of the elderly as a result of the disintegration of the family therein. It is true that this Western practice can be influenced by cultural, social, and individual considerations, seeing it either as a pragmatic approach to addressing the intricate requirements of aging populations or a deficiency in family support for the elderly. Yet, the philosophical contouring of these two societal norms are controversial. One is traditionally communitarian, while the other is materialistically and individualistically contractual. In an Arab context, however, similar institutions are out of the question. The average individual there, certainly, does not exist outside a vast web of social rituals and religious values; his existence is primarily socio-historical, and individual in the second place (Elmessiri 1979, 36). Put differently, the typical person's existence is deeply intertwined with social customs and religious beliefs, that neither individuality nor any materialist concerns could overcome.

Herd Immunity, *Homo Senex*, and Masked Eugenics

In terms of historical antecedents, the culture of modernity in the West presented great challenges and unrest in consistency with its underlying secular assumptions, its cultural and ideological agendas, and all sorts of justifications to put them on track.[2] Thus, the post-enlightenment scientific mindset deemed it permissible to subject the multitudes to voluntary deadly experimentation in the name of progress and pseudoscience, awash in its Neo-Darwinist misconceptions about humans as this chapter will demonstrate. Expectedly, this development culminated in Nazi genocide in Europe with the *Homo Europaeus* as the perfect model of racial superiority (Kuhl 1994, 17). The origins lie in eugenics, historically a Western flawed ideology that advocated for improving human genetics through selective breeding and sterilization, while it was often driven by misconceptions surrounding race, gender, and physical or mental abilities.

Covid-19 was another significant juncture in that long history of evolutionism and natural selection that cemented tolerant and passive confidence in nature as the new deity. Thus, quarantine, lockdown, partial containment, banning outdoors activities, implementing social distancing protocols stood in no manner compared to herd immunity as a drastic scientific measure against the pandemic.[3] The voluntary exposure of the populations to infection is grounded in the belief that epidemic termination depends on the changes in the properties of the infectious agent as it loses its virulence within a serial passage between vulnerable and immune segments of the population (Fine 1993, 266–267). The way the graying population, among other infirm groups, were abandoned unveils not only the health crisis of the contracting welfare state, but more incisively, the human deficiencies of Western society. Reminiscent of Nazi rhetoric, the attribute *homo senex* of the *Homo Europaeus*— treated like a *pariah*— has voluntarily been dispensed with in the name of a herd immunity heterodoxy. Alongside the deficiency of will to save human lives, the indiscriminate and dutiful universality of healthcare for all, which is a major Kantian principle, has been transgressed. Kant points out,

> that which refers to universal human inclinations and needs has a market price; that which, even without presupposing any need, is in accord with a certain taste, i.e., a satisfaction in the mere purposeless play of the powers of our mind, an affective price; but that which constitutes the condition under which alone something can be an end in itself does not have merely a relative worth, i.e., a price, but rather an inner worth, i.e., dignity. (2002, 52–53)

Abstaining from any measure which could alter a blind natural course based on a biased definition of the human essence, reduced to its nature/matter base, reflects the dehumanizing effect of the modern world in its Western formula.

Amid the pandemic, saving lives through healthcare provisions is no longer a moral obligation or a duty in the Kantian sense. Human dignity has not only been sacrificed to the market ethics but also transgressed in the name of scientific advancement. The plain truth is that the pandemic has exacerbated discrimination based on health conditions toward the infirm, disabled, elderly, or overweight. Immanuel Kant emphasizes that the promotion of happiness should not spring from inclination but from duty as a mandatory attribute of the rational being that the Enlightenment deified. Thus said,

> love as inclination cannot be commanded; but beneficence solely from duty, even when no inclination at all drives us to it, or even when natural and invincible disinclination resists, is practical and not pathological love, which lies in the will and not in the propensity of feeling, in the principles of action and not in melting sympathy; but the former alone can be commanded. (Kant 2002, 15)

During Covid-19, blind faith in scientific progress shelves any such ethical approach of human frailty. In the absence of a strong sense of duty toward one's fellow men, the scientist's humanness is rendered to nullity once the decision about who lives and who dies is made. To corroborate the idea that science without ethics is blind, Kant sees that

> [a]ll sciences have some practical part, consisting of the problems whether any end is possible for us and of imperatives about how it can be attained. These can therefore in general be called imperatives of skill. Whether the end is rational and good is not the question here, but only what one has to do in order to achieve them. The precepts for the physician, how to make his patient healthy in a well-grounded way, and for the poisoner, how to kill him with certainty, are to this extent of equal worth, since each serve to affect its aim perfectly. (2002, 31–32)

Undertaking their function in an efficient way, scientists could execute the task only from without, never from within, which calls for a detached state of mind or a mental and emotional distance *vis à vis* human experience. Thus, the scientific mindset becomes an agent of a dehumanizing naturalization that is rooted in the ultimate category of a deterministic nature-matter paradigm when it sacrifices duty and dedication to human sanctity to a degrading pragmatism, devoid of any moral qualms.

From the outset, voices within scientific circles and international health organizations could not refrain from calming the highly mediatized global public that large numbers of the population could build herd immunity through natural infection, while the vulnerable may constitute collateral damage in pursuit of that objective. The so-called Great Barrington Declaration (GBD), written by mainly "think tank" researchers, staunchly believed that by letting the virus run its normal course, the aim is to "reduce the considerable collateral damage for less vulnerable people who face more danger from lockdown than they do from COVID-19 infection."[4] Such bold statements are unethical seeing that it was enthused by economic motivations and profit-driven incentives. Reminiscent of "Useless eaters," as the Nazi phrase goes, people with such conditions are just "disposable human surplus" because they ceased to contribute anything to Western society (Elmessiri 1996, 46–47). Thus, priority was given to the mental and economic welfare of the most at the expense of the lost lives of the rest.

The idea of relying on natural infection to develop herd immunity, as was promoted by such bodies as the Great Barrington Declaration, entwines both the pseudo-scientific assumptions of Darwinism and the social dimensions of Nietzscheanism. Traditionally, Europe started to catalogue humans as either Nietzschean *supermen*—the powerful pole in Darwinian natural selection—that identify with imperialism, or *submen,* mainly functional people under the willpower of the *supermen* (Elmessiri 1997a, 27). By legitimizing such individualistic ideologies, "power and the will to power have become the only acceptable metaphysics and the only epistemological and ethical point of stability" (Elmessiri 1994, 406–407). Such decentering of man resulted in exposing him to the hegemony of the scientific mind and senses (Elmessiri 2002e, 209–210). In practice, there emerged "theories of evolution and decay [*Entartung*], the importance of heredity, and the possibility of race improvement—in short, the ideas of Darwin, Mendel, and Gallon— [that] were penetrating Western scientific thought and social life" (Kuhl 1994, 16). Western handling of a primarily medical crisis such as Covid-19 was another chapter of submitting elderly *submen* to a systematic extermination, indicative of Western recurrent transgression of the sanctity of human beings.

A related concept in this regard is eugenics, originally a veterinary concept. The idea is based on the sheer natural selection and survival of the fittest that served to perpetrate major atrocities by modernity's dark forces. And what is herd immunity but the incarnation of an aggressive Darwinism put into operation on humans. Historically, research ethics were first transgressed by scientific experts operating from major Western scientific bodies. Long before Nazi Germans adopted policies to improve the Aryan human stock and purify the Teutonic population against the race-mixing "contaminations" of immigrants from other races, eugenics as a laboratory practice dates to the beginning of the twentieth century. Germano-American connections through the "Pioneer Fund can help us understand Nazi race ideology and the results and implications of present-day race research as part of a shared history of scientific racism" (Kuhl 1994, 11). Charles Darwin regrets how,

> with savages, the weak in body or mind are soon eliminated; and those that survive commonly exhibit a vigorous state of health. We civilized men, on the other hand, do our utmost to check the process of elimination; we build asylums for the imbecile, the maimed, and the sick; we institute poor-laws; and our medical men exert their utmost skill to save the life of every one to the last moment. There is reason to believe that vaccination has preserved thousands, who from a weak constitution would formerly have succumbed . . . . Thus, the weak members of civilized societies propagate their kind. (1871, 281–282)

Removing such "impurities" from the white races' gene pool took eugenicists of the first world a series of international conferences, collaborative projects, and controversial research experimentation on humans. It started with the 300 participants in the International Congress of 1912 among whom was Leonard Darwin, son of the famous evolution theorist, Graham Bell, and Home Affairs secretary Winston Churchill (Kuhl 1994,14). The Second International Eugenics Congress was held in New York in 1921 without German racial hygienists in the aftermath of the First World War (Kuhl 1994, 18). Primary interwar link German scientist Geza von Hoffmann was astonished at American radicalism to implement legislated laws of sterilization of the "unfit," "feebleminded," and the mentally handicapped.[5] Thus,

> [t]he Commission of the American Genetic Association, headed by Harry H. Laughlin, proposed that the lowest 10 percent of the American population be sterilized. This extreme measure, never seriously considered for state legislation, was intended to "eradicate" the "inferior" members of the society over a time period spanning two generations. Despite his doubts concerning the feasibility of such measures, Hoffmann praised the proposal for accurately illustrating the extent to which sterilization needed to be implemented. (Kuhl 1994, 18)

The International Federation of Eugenics Organizations, replacing the Permanent International Eugenics Committee, was established in the late 1920s while the Third International Eugenics Congress was held in 1932, resulting in enlarging the scope of expertise, integrating other fields of knowledge, moving from pure eugenics to "applied eugenics," and legislating and adopting eugenics' principles by Western nations (Kuhl 1994, 21–22). This provides ample evidence about how initial violations of research ethics were perpetrated by esteemed scientific figures, operating from prominent Western scientific institutions.

Prior to the Nazis implementing negative eugenics on non-Germans, the annals of history are fraught with disreputable incidents perpetrated by unethical experimentation on humans mainly in the United States. Four decades of the Tuskegee Syphilis Study (1932–1972) is still fresh in the hearts and minds of the American Black community. On the premise that racial nervous resistance of Black Americans to the lethal venereal disease is arguably true, the experiment "draws attention to the power of racial theory to shape medical knowledge and to steer American medical researchers into an especially destructive undertaking" (Crenner 2012, 246). As Brandt puts it, the experiment was more concerned with "the pathology of racism than it did about the pathology of syphilis; more about the nature of scientific inquiry than the nature of the disease process" (1978, 27). The experiment itself offers abundant proof of how reverence on behalf of humanity and its moral defense can be undermined in pursuit of misguided pseudo-scientific advancement.

Another chapter where the sanctity of humanity and its moral shield have been transgressed is the Willowbrook Hepatitis Experiments in 1956, whereby children with intellectual disabilities were voluntarily infected, exploiting their disabilities and the disadvantaged social circumstances of their families for consent. In defense of the experiment, researchers claimed to observe natural infection in play and insisted their protocols were ethical (Rothman 1982, 6). Such experiments offer valuable insights into how far from natural such plight was, while it was a meticulously orchestrated outcome of a greatly stage-managed human intervention. Supposedly, "where the essential cause of a health problem is social deprivation, it is generally within the power of the research team to remedy the situation for their subjects. Hence, they cannot be 'observers' to a plight they could improve" (Rothman 1982, 7). Likewise, while the protection and rescue of the Covid-19 struck elderly were possible in Western retirement houses, letting them prey to natural infection questions Western ethical principles that guide modern clinical judgment and allegedly beneficial scientific research. Discrimination by age (the elderly), by baseline health condition and coerced consent (Willowbrook children with intellectual disabilities), or by socially and racially disadvantaged position (Tuskegee Syphilis contaminated Black men) proved real moral failures by Western scientists. The Nazi genocide stood as the paradigmatic secular moment of all times, seeing that it perpetrated the methodical extermination of millions in a rational and detached manner which makes it an essential current in Western civilization (Elmessiri 1997a, 13). Thus,

> if we place Nazism first in the broader context of the theories of racial inequality that spread in Europe in the second half of the 19th century and which formed the doctrinal basis of Western imperialism, and second, in the context of the systematic genocide of native Americans and the enslavement of native Africans by Westerners. If we do so, we will find that Nazism—labelled by many as a mere aberration from a humanistic Western civilisation—was actually a paradigmatic moment and part of an overall Western recurrent pattern, different from other similar phenomena only in degree not in kind. (Elmessiri 2006, 56)

At some point, the Western secular mind, embracing ideals of deterministic progress, showed a disinterest toward human vulnerability. The current pandemic emphasizes how persistently challenging Western medical ethics of balancing that progress with human needs are.

Relaunching the Economy, Big Pharma, and Vaccines for the Global South

Markedly, the symbolic drafting and signature of the GBD at the American Institute for Economic Research is eloquently evocative. Its signatories articulated a eugenic *rationale* to endorse opening the economy; favoring market ethics over people's lives. Doing so, especially in the neoliberal world to the detriment of containing the pandemic, interrogates the Western conception of the human being it once sought to overvalue. Among the manifestations of the collapse of the human order is the issue of rights and freedoms that have been emptied of their traditional content to advance a free economic subject. According to the *New York Times*, despite "having some of the toughest measures in the world, Italian authorities fumbled many of those steps early in the contagion—when it most mattered as they sought to preserve basic civil liberties as well as the economy."[6] Such distress calls about the economy and liberties amid the contagion are an indication of the hegemony of a wild anarchic capitalism that does not abide by any theory of value, except accumulating surpluses, insatiable profit-oriented ventures, and the well-being of the few.

Prior to vaccine availability, with unprecedented infection peaks worldwide, and a misguided herd immunity, the risks of opening the economy reflect the impact of capitalist processes on the very existence of the Western Man. As an absolute contractual modern society, radical developments led to the emergence of an atypical version of Adam Smith's archetypal *homo economicus* with his sole inducement to accumulate material riches or else the erogenous man with his uninhibited drive for satisfaction (Elmessiri 2002d, 375). Elmessiri contends that "when we say that the world (humanity and nature) is subject completely to the laws of nature," it means that "Man is defined either in terms of production or reproduction" (1996, 5). Modern-day society's irrationality as a whole resides in its destructive productivity to allegedly answer human needs and faculties (Marcuse 1964, xi). The one-dimensional man's agency, free will, and capabilities have been exhausted in the name of economic advancement and an intermittent consumption. In his identification of the traditional forces that quarreled over Man's ultimate exploitation despite the possibility to qualify his life conditions, Marcuse continues,

> the union of growing productivity and growing destruction; the brinkmanship of annihilation; the surrender of thought, hope, and fear to the decisions of the powers that be; the preservation of misery in the face of unprecedented wealth constitute the most impartial indictment—even if they are not the *raison d'être* of this society but only its by-product, its sweeping rationality, which propels efficiency and growth, is itself irrational. (1964, xiiv)

Accordingly, denying him his dignity, self-worth, and security in the name of progress, this dismissal of Man entails the rise of a new order where the state just devours society instead of serving it. It indicates the eclipse of what is solidary and organic by what is mechanistic and contractual, where the human factor's value, if any, is of a secondary or tertiary concern.

Amid this degeneracy into a pro-nature, pro-matter, and anti-human paradigm, Western materialist monism tends toward inventiveness to sustain its reductionist view of the world. Marcuse explores the latest stages of the repressive ideological utilization of Man in the technologically advanced society wherewith "Men, in following their own reason, follow those who put their reason to profitable use" (1941, 148). The durability is usually on the side of the natural order and its highly rational and contractual processes while social forces and the human subject are the ones who should grapple with adjustments to it to suit their coercive anxieties and urgent demands. Marcuse calls it "non-terroristic economic-technical coordination which operates through the manipulation of needs by vested interests," within a modern capitalist mode of production and a system of distribution compatible with a "pluralism" of "countervailing powers" (1964, 5). In the final stand, humanity not only digresses to a position lower than that of nature/matter, but is still at the mercy of its assiduously innovative ways and means of exploitation.

Remarkably, Western thought no longer sanctions the autonomy of the human factor but instead turns Man into an entity that is subjected to materialist manipulation to serve sustain his one-dimensionality. The Enlightenment ideals' plan, whereby the world started to be homocentric, promoting humanity's complete emancipation through the negation of its limited moral existence generated a new definition of the allegedly free subject whose "performance is motivated, guided, and measured by standards external to him." The aim is to reach goals "which he did not set" (Marcuse 1941, 142). Marcuse argues that irrespective of how satisfied of his needs the Western Man is, those needs remain "products of a society whose dominant interest demands repression" (1964, 7). It is a willful theft by the social forces at work in the totalitarian advanced industrial society through the exercises of authority that organizes, manipulates, controls not only his social relationships but his productivity in compliance with its dictates of standardized control, production, and consumption (Marcuse 1941, 146). Ultimately, pragmatism or the disciplined adaptability to a wild material life has been provided with all what sustains them in the Western Man's stead. This entails deserting the fundamental Adamic tradition, universally acclimatized to communitarian relations of symbiosis, solidarity, and organicity.

In line with Zygmunt Bauman's theses, moving from "solid" to "liquid" modernity has generated new societal dynamics and the corresponding repositioning of the human element by and through them. The philosopher of liquidity sees in that "an infinity of improvements, with no 'final state' in sight and none desired" (Bauman 2012, ix). The plight out of eclipsing or weakening agency comes from how much subservient to economy, politics have grown to be (Bauman 2011, 53–54). The immediate harm is "to harness popular consent for neoliberal stripping back of social protections" (Coleman and Mullin-McCandlish 2021, 171). This overtaking empowered originally individualistic actants in world business, financial systems, banking authorities, and the monetary funds who engage in a "'polycentrism' of action on a planet integrated by a dense web of interdependencies" (Bauman 2012, xiv). In the age of Covid-19, big pharma laboratories thrived as lobbying groups, offering exclusive services, competitively and hegemonically operating on a transnational level and primely motivated by capitalistic greed instead of unconditionally rescuing a distressed humanity. No wonder, "the reason we have the vaccine 'success' is because of capitalism, because of greed my friends" unashamedly observed PM Boris Johnson at a Zoom meeting with Tory backbenchers on the vaccine push (Allegretti and Elgot 2021). Such an inflammatory rhetoric reflects the growing public discontent with the true motives and practices of pharmaceutical key players amid the pandemic.

Having in mind this disorienting outcome where the traditional points of referentiality are lost, Bauman expresses skepticism regarding the potential for redemption. He claims that under the aegis of the contractual society, community is the paradise lost and "the kind of world which is not, regrettably, available to us—but which we would dearly wish to inhabit and which we hope to repossess" (2001, 3). Social structures that determine individual choices, and institutions that guarantee a set of accepted habits, patterns of behavior, and frames of reference for human actions are short-lived or simply nonexistent. Within this state of unrest, appeasing individual suffering is no longer a societal priority while the dangers arising from fluctuations in the labor, competitiveness, and commodity markets are maintained. In other words, freelance is given to the ephemeral against the stable, need is dethroned by desire, necessity lends the way for pragmatism and profit-making while chaos engulfs all (Bauman 2012, 212). For Bauman, such degraded human essence's ability to convalesce seems out of reach.

Amid the pandemic, disparities were strongly sensed in supposedly non-liberal or less liberal countries in contrast to the situation in the neoliberal West that lay claim to advanced health and economic systems. Heavily investing in its healthcare systems, China's neutralization of rights and liberties and sacrificing the economy helped in times of collective emergency once the power of the panopticon state was regained to contain the pandemic (Chalk 2021, 92). As of the organic symbiotic community type, "the least neoliberal countries in the world have come through the pandemic in better shape" (Chalk 2021, 91). If anything should be pointed out as accountable for any failure to handle the pandemic in major ultra-neoliberal countries, it is anarchic global capitalism, which "both promotes and veils mass harms to populations" (Coleman and Mullin-McCandlish 2021, 170). Certainly, the logic of responsive compassion on the part of most non-Western countries' officials spared their populations the worst.

Remarkably, the authoritarian, the democratic, and the neoliberal responses coped differently with the pandemic. Unlike non-liberal countries, where there is always a difference between the human priority approach and the economic priority approach, the United Kingdom, in its efforts to restore fiscal discipline, has implemented nearly a decade of austerity, which has blunted its ability to respond to the coronavirus. The United States, instead of implementing universal healthcare, has the highest defense spending on the planet. The Trump administration knew in January 2017 that America would be unable to meet the demands of a contagious disease outbreak, yet he chose to ignore the report, treating healthcare as a private good. The strongest approaches have come from the democratic, non-neoliberal approaches of New Zealand, Germany, and Taiwan, which have not needed to increase the power of the surveillance states because they continue to treat health care as a public rather than private good (James Chalk 2021, 97).

Clearly, the countries which did well have strong reservations *apropos* freeing vital sectors of public order and safety such as healthcare to economic and financial speculations. One of the most raucous declarations that marked the pandemic, according to *The Guardian*, is governor of Texas Dan Patrick's bold statement that people should die than put economy to peril (Beckett 2020). It is an upgrade from "letting die" to "making die," whereby certain populations were deemed "not only as disposable, but in fact only valuable when dead" (Darian-Smith 2021, 62). The logic here is free market and profit stripped of any value, except for the values of capital, while considering the vulnerable as "the crowd [which] is thus the antithesis of the 'community' and the perverted realization of individuality" (Marcuse 1941, 150). Countries that fared well in the crisis clearly sacrificed privatizing healthcare to safeguard public safety.

The chances of the third world to get their share of vaccines on behalf of their populations is another major issue. Struck by low-income countries having not yet received a single dose while wealthier ones almost inoculated their entire population, UN secretary-general António Guterres reminds "we see many examples of vaccine nationalism and vaccine hoarding in wealthier countries—as well as continued side deals with manufacturers that undermine access for all." [7] According to an Oxfam report, the alliance of nearly seventy organizations and UNAIDS attributes lower shares of vaccine to the Global South to monopolies and excessive prices that firms akin to Pfizer, BioNTech, and Moderna charged their clients. According to Anna Marriott, Oxfam's Health Policy Manager, they are "the most lethal cases of profiteering in history."[8] Inequity concerns "hoarding of surplus vaccines, blocking shipments to other countries and orders from them, and stymieing countries such as India and Africa to bypass intellectual property regimes to develop Covid diagnostic kits and cheap vaccines" (Kampmark and Kurečić, 2022, 15). The rationale behind such chauvinism is that vaccine donations to ease global inequality should ensure they cover wealthy states' own populations first (Kampmark and Kurečić, 2022, 10). Trapped in a framework of deserving vs. undeserving, humanity becomes a victim of its own categories. Another setback is the international rush to secure doses through bidding wars to monopolize an originally life-saving technology. Ostensibly, Americans seem to prioritize self-interest out of patriotic capitalism instead of vaccine supply out of humanitarian cooperation (Kampmark and Kurečić 2022, 11). According to *Die Welt*'s business correspondent Anja Ettel, Trump is said to have tried to lure German vaccine provider CureVac. Despite the company's denial, a lot remains unclear along a series of dismissals and changes in management. Dismissing any lingering doubts failed when Chancellor Angela Merkel declared the issue as "solved" in a press conference. All these further boosted mysteries around the case, points out Anja Ettel.

The international press also reported how some countries of the first world resorted to piracy in international air to steal medical equipment bound for other countries. Thinking that all rights are theirs without being bound by duties, Americans bluntly sequestered a shipment of 200,000 face masks destined for Germany at the Bangkok airport. Berlin Secretary of Interior Andreas Geisel qualified it an "act of modern piracy." According to Reuters reporter, "Allies of the United States from Europe to South America have complained about 'Wild West' tactics they say Washington has employed to outbid or block shipments of medical supplies to original buyers."[9] The US firm that produced them for German police refrained from the deal under a law prohibiting the export of medical supplies invoked by Trump: "We need these items immediately for domestic use. We have to have them."[10] Unauthorized diversions of medical equipment by supposedly developed nations raise concerns about equitable access to those resources.

Another significant incident indicative of the notion of "the crowd" dethroning that of "community" is how EU failed to succor one of its founding members whose populations were highly stricken by the pandemic. Alternatively, Italy, with all its history, European affiliation, and ancient heritage, humbly received the queue of Cuban doctors with warm and deserved applause, in recognition and gratitude for the support, humanitarian aid, and most importantly unconditional assistance coming from an overseas third world country. Surprisingly, EU countries, while abandoning each other, extended their hand to the "oft-maligned" Chinese for assistance which was unconceivable prior to Covid-19 outbreak.

Conclusion

This chapter cogitates major ethical and philosophical dilemmas that underwhelmed humanity amid the outbreak of different variants of the new coronavirus in its global echoes. Regardless of skeptics or conspiracists, the way the pandemic was handled raises fundamental questions about humanity's true essence and the previously stable ground beneath our conception of the Man of Enlightenment. The endeavor is to come to grips with the profound challenges that have emerged amid the global spread of Covid-19 and how it unveils the value of human existence within a series of similar paradigmatic secular moments throughout Western intellectual history. In the crucible of the pandemic, fundamental reconsiderations regarding the very core of human nature are reignited within the framework of a Western thought that initially sermonized human sanctity over any other worldly or otherworldly concerns, advancing the individual with reason illuminating his path to a cherished progress. Despite the ignited revolutions, paradigm-shifting intellectual breakthroughs, and undeniable World-altering technological advances that the West contributed to the shareholding corporation called human civilization, the pandemic stripped naked accompanying inequalities, and questioned social justice and the global common good, fervidly exalted in Western political philosophy. The collective crisis is an indication of the fall of the human *donnée* on the path to that aborted progress, "where all aspects of human activity become autonomous, self-validating, and self-referential, outside the individual's grip and choice" as Elmessiri puts it (1996, 47). Prioritizing profit-making at the expense of saving millions of lives put to the test the first world's humanitarian response and its alleged preparedness to crises of such magnitudes. The crisis interrogates the value of human existence in the face of a wild anarchic capitalism, and a Darwinian pseudo-scientific *rationale* that does not abide by any theory of value. It also divulges an anti-human element within an anarchic materialist context where scientific and technological progress are sought after at any human cost.

Notes

1 Elmessiri's projected model to map the secular mind in the West goes above the fragmentary process in dealing with human phenomena in a way that the range of isolated incidents hides some interconnectedness and homogeneity that Western models do not account for. This is what Elmessiri refers to as the paradigmatic secular sequence, the paradigmatic moment, and the paradigmatic figure. Elmessiri supposes that his model secures independence from concrete history, overlooks details, and skips sequences in look for coherent structures with great classifying and generalizing powers (1997a, 231). He also calls it a "discovered relationship" or a "paradigmatic moment" (اللحظة النماذجية الكاشفة الدالة) (El-Messiri1996, 43) wherein the secular sequence unfolds. This does not mean, however, that Elmessiri's model is timeless; rather, it unfolds through different historical junctures as a coherent whole (El-Messiri1996, 46).

2 In the name of progress, Western civilization has committed numerous atrocities throughout human history, often rationalized through various means. These major atrocities include the transatlantic slave trade, colonial genocide and territorial expansion massacres, world wars, economic exploitation, social and political suppression, cultural imperialism, and even environmental degradation. Common justifications for these actions have included the civilizing mission, manifest destiny doctrine, scientific racism and social Darwinism, progress, preemptive war for national security, military hegemony to enhance prestige, the balance of power, all types of religious justification, and multiple political ideologies to support them.

3 Herd immunity was first practiced in veterinary research on cows in interwar America (Eichornand Potter, 1917).

4 GBD https://gbdeclaration.org/frequently-asked-questions/ (Accessed January 1, 2023).

5 In the United States, Indiana was the first to illegally perform eugenic sterilization of the mentally handicapped in 1899. In 1909, followed California and Connecticut with similar measures. In 1911, Nevada, Iowa, and New Jersey did the same. In 1912, it was the turn of New York while, Kansas, Michigan, North Dakota, and Oregon also legislated sterilization laws in 1913 (Kuhl 1994, 17).

6 In 2020, the leader of the governing Democratic Party Nicola Zingaretti advertised a picture of himself in the local press clinking wine glasses for "an aperitivo in Milan," calling on Italians "not to change our habits." Horowitz et al. (2020).

7 António Guterres's Statement on the COVID-19 Pandemic (2021).

8 Oxfam (2021).

9 Tanakasempipat (2020).

10 Hackenbroich et al. (2020).

References

Allegretti, A. and J. Elgot. "Covid, 'Greed' and Capitalism behind Vaccine Success, Johnson Tells MPs." *The Guardian,* March 24, 2021. https,//www.theguardian.com/politics/2021/mar/23/greed-and-capitalism-behind-jab-success-boris-johnson-tells-mps (Accessed May 12, 2023).

António Guterres's Statement on the COVID-19 Pandemic. One Year On "Only Together can we End this Pandemic and Recover." March 11, 2021. https,//www.un.org/en/coronavirus/only-together-can-we-end-pandemic-and-recover (Accessed July 3, 2023).

Bauman, Zygmunt. *Community, Seeking Safety in an Insecure World.* Cambridge: Polity Press, 2001.

Bauman, Zygmunt. *Collateral Damage, Social Inequalities in a Global Age.* Cambridge: Polity Press, 2011.

Bauman, Zygmunt. *Liquid Modernity.* Cambridge: Polity Press, 2012.

Beckett, L. "Older People would Rather die than Let COVID-19 Harm US Economy, Texas Official." *The Guardian,* March 24, 2020. https,//www.theguardian.com/world/2020/mar/24/older-people-would-rather-die-than-let-COVID-19-lockdown-harm-us-economy-texas-official-dan-patrick (Accessed July 2, 2023).

Belsky, Janet K. *The Psychology of Aging : Theory, Research, and Interventions.* Pacific Grove, Calif. London : Brooks/Cole Publishing Co, 3rd ed, 1999.

Berman, M. *All that is Solid Melts into Air, The Experience of Modernity.* London and New York: Verso, 1983.

Brandt, Allan M. "Racism and Research, The Case of the Tuskegee Syphilis Study." *The Hastings Center Report* 8, no. 6 (December 1978): 21–29.

Chalk, James. "Neoliberalism and Personal Freedoms during COVID-19." *Journal of Global Faultlines* 8, no. 1 (2021): 91–99.

Coleman, R. and B. Mullin-McCandlish. "The Harms of State, Free-Market Common Sense and COVID-19." *State Crime Journal* 10, no. 1 (2021): 170–188.

Crenner, Christopher. "The Tuskegee Syphilis Study and the Scientific Concept of Racial Nervous Resistance." *Journal of the History of Medicine and Allied Sciences* 67, no. 2 (April 2012): 244–280.

Darian-Smith, E. "Dying for the Economy, Disposable People and Economies of Death in the Global North." *State Crime Journal* 10, no. 1 (2021): 61–79.

Darwin, Charles. *The Descent of Man and Selection in Relation to Sex.* 2nd ed. London: John Murray, 1871.

Eichorn, A. and G.M. Potter. *Contagious Abortion of Cattle.* Farmer's Bulletin 790. Washington, DC: United States Department of Agriculture, 1917.

Elliott, Kevin. "Biomedical Ethics, Public-Health Risk Assessment, and the Naturalistic Fallacy." *Public Affairs Quarterly* 16, no. 4 (Oct., 2002): 351–376.

El-Messiri, Abdelwahab. *Al-Firdaws al-Arḍī, Dirāsāt wa Inṭibā'āt 'an al-Ḥaḍārah al-Amrīkīyah al-Ḥadīthah* (The earthly paradise, studies and reflections on contemporary American civilization). Beirut: al-Mu'assasah al-'Arabīyah lil-Dirāsāt wa al-Nashr, 1979.

El-Messiri, Abdelwahab. "The Imperialist Epistemological Vision." *The American Journal of Islamic Social Sciences (AJISS)* 11, no. 3 (1994): 403–415.

El-Messiri, Abdelwahab. "Parables of Freedom and Necessity, The Rising Levels of Secularization as Manifested in Two Literary Works." *The American Journal of Islamic Social Sciences* (*AJISS*) 13, no. 1 (1996): 42–58.

El-Messiri, Abdelwahab. *A-ṣuhyūniyyah wa an-nāziyyah wa nihāyat at-tārīkh* (Zionism, Nazism and the End of History), 5th ed. Cairo: Dar El-Shurouk, 1997a.

El-Messiri, Abdelwahab. "The Dance of the Pen, the Play of the Sign, A Study in the Relationship between Modernity, Immanence, and Deconstruction." *The American Journal of Islamic Social Sciences* (*AJISS*) 14, no. 1 (1997b): 1–12.

El-Messiri, Abdelwahab. *Fikr ḥarakat al-istināra wa tanāqodatūh* (Enlightenment thought and its contradictions). Cairo: Dar Nahdet Misr, 1998.

El-Messiri, Abdelwahab. *Al- 'ālam min Manḍur Gharbi* (The world from a Western perspective). Cairo: Dār Al-Hilāl, Kitāb Al-Hilāl, 2000.

El-Messiri, Abdelwahab. *Al-lughah wa al-majāz bayna at-tawḥīd wa wiḥdat al-wujūd* (Language and metaphor between monotheism and pantheism), 3rd ed. Cairo: Dar El-Shurouk, 2002a.

El-Messiri, Abdelwahab. *Al-Jamat al-wazifiyah al-yahūdiyah, Namūdhaj tafsīrī jadīd* (The Jewish functional groups, a new interpretive model), 3rd ed. Cairo: Dar El-Shorouk, 2002d.

El-Messiri, Abdelwahab. *Epistemological Bias in the Physical and Social Sciences.* London and Washington: The International Institute of Islamic Thought, 2006.

Ettel, Anja. "Was bei CureVac nach Trumps Avancen passierte, wirft Fragen auf." *Die Welt*, March 17, 2020. https,//www.welt.de/wirtschaft/article206620503/CureVac-Ungereimtheiten-um-Hersteller-von-CoronaImpfstoff.html (Accessed July 3, 2023).

Fine, Paul E. M. "Herd Immunity, History, Theory, Practice." *Epidemiologic Reviews by the* Johns Hopkins University School of Hygiene and Public Health 15, no. 2 (1993): 265–302.

Hackenbroich, J., J. Shapiro, and T. Varma, T. "Health Sovereignty, How to Build a Resilient European Response to Pandemics." *European Council on Foreign Relations*, 2020. http,//www.jstor.org/stable /resrep25376 (Accessed March 10, 2023).

Horowitz, Jason, Emma Bubola, and Elisabetta Povoledo. "Italy, Pandemic's New Epicenter, Has Lessons for the World." *New York Times*, March 21, 2020. https,//www.nytimes.com/2020/03/21/world/europe/italy-coronavirus-center-lessons.html.

Kampmark, B. and P. Kurečić. "Vaccine Nationalism, Competition, EU Parochialism, and COVID-19." *Journal of Global Faultlines* 9, no. 1 (2022): 9–20.

Kant, Immanuel, et al. *Groundwork for the Metaphysics of Morals*. Edited by Allen W. Wood, Yale University Press, 2002.

Kuhl, Stephen. *The Nazi Connection Eugenics, American Racism, and German National Socialism*. New York and Oxford: Oxford University Press, 1994.

Lal, A., N. A. Erondu, D. L. Heymann, G. Gitahi, and R. Yates "Fragmented Health Systems In COVID-19, Rectifying the Misalignment between Global Health Security and Universal Health Coverage." *The Lancet* 397 (2021): 61–7.

Marcuse, Herbert. *One Dimensional Man; Studies in the Ideology of Advanced Industrial Society*. Boston: Beacon Press, 1964.

Marcuse, Herbert. "Some Social Implications of Modern Technology." In Andrew Arato and Eike Gebhardt (Eds.), *The Essential Frankfurt School Reader*, 138–162. Oxford: Basil Blackwell, 1978 [1941].

Ogden, Lydia L. and Kathleen Adams. "Poorhouse to Warehouse, Institutional Long-Term Care in the United States." *Publius* 39, no. 1 (2009): 138–163.

Oxfam. July 29, 2021. https,//www.oxfam.org/en/press-releases/vaccine-monopolies-make-cost-vaccinating-world-against-covid-least-5-times-more (Accessed May 12, 2023).

Remuzzi, Andrea and Giuseppe Remuzzi. "COVID-19 and Italy: What Next?" *The Lancet* 395, no. 10231 (2020): 1225–1228.

Rothman, D.J. "Were Tuskegee & Willowbrook 'Studies in Nature'?" *Hastings Center Report* 12, no. 2 (1982): 5–7.

Tanakasempipat, Patpicha. "Accused of 'piracy', U.S. Denies Diverting Masks Bound for Germany." *Reuters*, April 6 2020. https,//www.reuters.com/article/us-health-coronavirus-masks-idUSKBN21O0Y0 (Accessed June 2, 2023).

4

Denied Personhood

The Necropolitical Production of Disposability in Mediterranean Migration

Rachid Benharrousse

Introduction

Roberto Esposito's concept of the *dispositif of the Person* offers a compelling perspective to dissect the urgent and intricate dynamics of the Mediterranean migration crisis. This framework, which delves into the interplay between individuality, society, and power, is especially pertinent when scrutinizing the perceptions and treatment of irregular migrants (Esposito, 2012). In the context of Mediterranean migration, the dispositif of the Person categorizes certain migrants as disposable "living things" devoid of biopolitical potential. In contrast, others from the Global North are normalized as rights-bearing persons. The concept of immunity, which denotes the protective boundaries individuals establish to safeguard their identity and autonomy, is systematically denied to these migrants. They are often stripped of the rights and privileges that allow them to establish a distinct existence within European societies (Esposito, 2011). The notion of community is manipulated to exclude these migrants, positioning them outside the sphere of those whose lives are deemed valuable and worthy of protection and immunity.

The fluid and evolving nature of the Person's dispositif, as Esposito underscores, is demonstrated in the shifting policies and attitudes toward Mediterranean migrants. Historical, cultural, and political contexts shape how these migrants are perceived and managed, reflecting the contingent nature of personhood that Esposito describes (Esposito, 2012). For instance, the intensification of border controls and the criminalization of irregular migration can be seen as manifestations of the dispositif of the Person's adaptation to maintain neocolonial power dynamics. By applying Esposito's framework to the Mediterranean migration crisis, we can critically interrogate how the neoliberal paradigm, colonial legacies, and geopolitical considerations interact to shape the treatment of these migrants, often relegating them to a status of disposability.

Historicizing Mediterranean Migration

The Spanish-Moroccan border, particularly the enclaves of Ceuta and Melilla, represents a critical point in Mediterranean migration dynamics. Since the late 1990s, unauthorized boat migrants have been a pressing issue in Moroccan-Spanish relations, with routes diversifying to include departures from Southern Morocco and West Africa (Ferrer-Gallardo, 2008; Carling, 2007). Eliminating internal Schengen border controls in 1995 has further emphasized the Spanish-African border's role in regulating migration flows into Europe (Geddes, 2005). Sub-Saharan migrants have become half of the boat migrants intercepted along the Spanish coasts after departing from Morocco or "Western (Moroccan) Sahara" (Hernández-Carretero and Carling, 2012). Because it became much more expensive and challenging to access Europe through unauthorized means, Sub-Saharan migrants are becoming immigrants in North Africa rather than perceiving it as a means of clandestinity. However, most of these immigrants in North Africa lack the necessary finances to go to Europe or return to their country of origin, which propels them to live in impoverished circumstances (Ikuteyijo, 2014; de Haas, 2008) while seeking legal status in Morocco through the New Migration Policy inaugurated in 2013 by King Mohammed VI.

First, migrants who successfully cross the border "illegally" and without authorization become automatically "illegal" residents within Europe without rights or a right to rights (De Genova, 2002). The primary method for this entry into Spain from Africa has been small-scale smuggling in *pateras* (small wooden boats made primarily for fishing) (Carling, 2007). Others become "illegal" residents after overstaying a visa or another permit, while a third group becomes irregular residents after failing to return following an expulsion order (Düvell, 2011). Accordingly, unless the undocumented migrant leaves the host country, there are two ways of becoming documented: regularization and expulsion. The former is the most important in Spain and other Southern European countries, requiring proof of entry and a specified date in the past (Levinson, 1994). Of course, the unauthorized entries intercepted at the border are rejected and returned; this applies even to authorized migrants deemed inadmissible by the immigration officers (Spijkerboer, 2007). Most are denied entry because they are suspected of overstaying their visas, while others arrive with forged or insufficient documents, or without sufficient finances.

Certain unauthorized migrants enter Europe through fraudulent immigration officers, which resists border and state binaries because they become neither documented nor illegal (Triandafyllidou and Ambrosini, 2011). If the unauthorized migrant is apprehended after crossing the border or applies for asylum, they would enter a time-limited period during which their presence in the country is tolerated until their claim is examined or their expulsion is prepared (Düvell, 2011). Further, the return from within a country's territory to the country of origin is much more complicated than rejection at the border since it requires the country of origin's willingness to allow the "illegal" return (Gibney, 2008). This poses a severe challenge for migration management, particularly for countries experiencing unauthorized maritime immigration, which lacks a fixed route per se (Carrera, 2007). Accordingly, states seek to intercept boat migrants at sea and prevent them from reaching the country's territory (Pugh, 2004). For this reason, most migrants deliberately expose themselves to danger so that they can be rescued and taken ashore rather than returned to their countries (Spijkerboer, 2007).

Moroccans are the primary group among unauthorized immigrants through the Ceuta and Melilla borders and the Strait of Gibraltar (de Haas, 2008). During 2003, the population of legal Moroccan residents grew, with almost five persons for every Moroccan boat migrant intercepted along the coast (Carling, 2007). Spanish and EU authorities have taken measures to control unauthorized immigration for two primary reasons: to reduce the number of unauthorized residents in the EU and to expedite the expulsion of successful "illegal" residents (Geddes, 2005). To this end, Spain has taken several steps to dissuade would-be migrants from Morocco, whether native or transit(Ferrer-Gallardo, 2008). Also, it has pressured the Moroccan authorities to strengthen border controls, introduce stricter visa requirements for Sub-Saharan Africans, and obstruct human smuggling (Carling and Hernández-Carretero, 2011). This has been done through the European Neighborhood Policy and the Euro-Mediterranean Partnership programs (Lavenex and Uçarer, 2004).

Further, control measures include the case-by-case processing of apprehended migrants before the maximum detention period expires. In Spain, "illegals" arrested based on "illegal" entry or residence can be detained for up to three days. If their nationality is identified, the expulsion process is initiated, and they remain detained for up to forty days. Suppose their nationality is not determined and their expulsion has been unanswered by the country of origin for up to forty days. In that case, they are released with an expulsion order, which makes their stay illegal, yet they cannot be "removed" from the country (De Genova, 2002). During 2002 and 2003, only about a quarter of all expulsions were carried out due to difficulties in bilateral relations. However, the released migrants had expulsion orders that became impossible to execute (Carling, 2007; Buoli, 2014). The number of remaining migrants has exceeded 66,000, almost twice the number apprehended for illegal entry along the coast during the same years (González-Enríquez, 2009).

Spain has put much effort into facilitating the readmission of migrants to either transit countries or countries of origin (Cassarino, 2007). Spain has signed a readmission agreement with Morocco, under which Morocco must readmit all migrants who entered Spain illegally through Morocco, regardless of nationality (Cassarino, 2010). This agreement has been in effect since 1992. While Morocco has respected the readmission of Moroccans, the return of Sub-Saharan Africans has been problematic, especially because Morocco claims there is little evidence that Sub-Saharan Africans departed from Morocco (Collyer, 2007). This made Morocco avoid the agreement without breaching it. Yet, in October 2003, the Moroccan government agreed to readmit non-Moroccans who were arrested on pateras led by a Moroccan (Carling, 2007). This has strengthened the process of returning unauthorized migrants and placing them outside the EU, without the difficulties surrounding expulsion (Boswell, 2003).

The increasing number of fatalities further complicates migration control alongside the Spanish-African borders (Carling, 2007). During 2003 and 2004, twenty-one known boat accidents with over ten deaths added to the complicated difficulties surrounding surveillance and control (Spijkerboer, 2007). The vast majority of deaths in this area are drowning accidents, especially since most clandestine migrants are ordered to swim a long distance from the shore to allow the smuggler to escape the authorities (Triandafyllidou, 2010). Most migrants are either unable to swim or are caught in the currents. However, these are not the only dangers to which unauthorized migrants are exposed. The most dangerous situations arise during rescue or interception operations conducted by the Guardia Civil (Ferrer-Gallardo, 2008). The pateras are extremely unstable because of their heavy loads and poor construction. It is not unusual for pateras to carry twenty-five passengers over almost 90 km through the route to the Canary Islands (Carling, 2007). Because the patera is boarding so many migrants, any commotion can lead to their downfall; further, the Guardia Civil is not equipped to conduct large-scale rescues because their purpose is coastal surveillance and the fight against drug smuggling (Godenau, 2014). The Guardia Civil *rescues* only a handful of drowned migrants because of their inadequacy in these operations.

Motor failure is also a common issue, especially on long journeys. On the Strait of Gibraltar, pateras risk colliding with larger vessels or capsizing on the journey (Carling and Hernández-Carretero, 2011). Yet, on the route to the Canary Islands, pateras that do experience a breakdown can go unsighted for weeks. In recent years, many pateras have been sighted by accident and rescued (Godenau, 2014). In one of these cases, in February 2001, a patera was sighted by a fishing boat and rescued approximately 120 km south of the Canary Islands after two weeks. When the engine broke down halfway to Fuerteventura, the smugglers and two Moroccans were picked up by another patera, leaving eighteen Sub-Saharan Africans to drift. By the time of the rescue, twelve of them had died (Carling, 2007). Toxic gas, which is produced by the pateras around seawater near the boat, is hazardous when unauthorized migrants are forced to swim. Several migrants would suffocate at sea, as well as migrants who are hidden in cargo, sealed containers, and lorries (Spijkerboer, 2007).

The Spanish-African border remains a focal point for migration flows and complex bilateral relations at different levels: between Spain and Morocco, between Southern Europe and the Maghreb, and between the European Union and Africa (Geddes, 2005). The other issues surrounding Moroccan-Spanish bilateral relations, such as fishing rights, the Spanish enclaves, and the Moroccan Sahara, are furthering tensions between the two countries (Gillespie, 2006). The latter attempted to deepen cooperation, but accusations of collusion with smugglers, delays in developing SIVE, and complacency with the migration policy have become increasingly apparent, making it clear that there can be no technologically driven unilateral solution to the challenges of unauthorized migration (Carrera, 2007). This is highly the case because, as aforementioned, Spain attempts to prevent unauthorized migrants from arriving in Europe; yet, upon their arrival, their return highly depends on political priorities and resource commitments within Spain and the agreement of the country of transit and origin (Cassarino, 2007). However, there have been claims that Morocco has deliberately allowed large numbers of Sub-Saharan Africans and Moroccans to illegally cross toward the Canary Islands to stop their support for self-determination in the Moroccan Sahara (de Haas, 2008). The perception of migrants as "illegal" or "unauthorized" stems from this historical relationship, setting the stage for their treatment as less-than-human subjects and reinforcing the disposability of Mediterranean migrants.

Policy as Disposability: Necropolitics and Personhood

The Mediterranean Sea has tragically become a graveyard for countless irregular migrants attempting to reach Europe in search of safety, opportunity, personhood, and a better life (Lutterbeck, 2006). The latter is based on a dominant belief in Europe as *European Heaven,* wherein life is more accessible, meritocracy is evident, democracy is structured, and opportunity is abundant (Collyer, 2007). Yet, to reach this utopian space of European Heaven, irregular migrants must undertake a journey on overcrowded inflatable boats (Butler, 2019: 10), "burning" their documents and risking their lives. The treacherous journey across the Mediterranean has claimed the lives of thousands, with the relentless smuggling networks exacerbating the peril faced by these desperate, impersonal subjects (Sassen, 2016: 25). The statistics surrounding migrant deaths in the Mediterranean Sea reveal a disturbing reality. According to the International Organization for Migration (IOM), over the past decade, more than 20,000 migrants have lost their lives while attempting to cross the Mediterranean (Weiss, 2018: 45). These numbers, however, only represent the documented cases, and the actual death toll is believed to be significantly higher, as many incidents go unreported and bodies are often never recovered (Spijkerboer, 2007). The death toll has been rising year after year, reflecting a tragic failure to address the underlying causes and provide adequate assistance to those in need (Harvey, 2020: 15). Hence, because the irregular migrant is not European, the EU "chooses" to be blind to the steady and continuous rise of deaths in the Mediterranean (De Genova, 2017). In 2016 alone, the deadliest year on record, over 5,000 individuals perished in their attempts to cross the Mediterranean (Brown, 2018: 25).

The Mediterranean tragedy is perceived as a *natural* outcome of the neoliberal constitution of the Global South as economically inferior to the Global North and irregular migrants as living things (Mbembe, 2003). First, subjects from the Global South are perceived as naturally seeking out the Global North due to high unemployment rates (Castles, 2010). This further feeds into the logic of the global neoliberal order, assuming that the need to migrate became evident only when would-be migrants became unemployed. Under this logic, the EU has launched multiple programs and initiatives to "help" the Mediterranean countries reduce poverty and unemployment, while pushing for other changes through Structural Adjustment Programs. These programs further the already evident perception of European countries as *superior* and, naturally, subjects "should" seek Europe (Bigo, 2002). The European Neighborhood Policy (ENP) is the latest framework through which Europe seeks to "advance" the economies of Southern Mediterranean countries through aid (Del Sarto and Schumacher, 2005). This speaks to the *naturalized* order in which Europe helps the ex-colonies, irrespective of the colonial history through which they made and continue to make their current wealth (Bhambra, 2016). Hence, the Euro-Mediterranean Partnership was inaugurated in 1995 to advance political cooperation, economic development, and cultural understanding between European and MENA countries (Gillespie, 2008). This and other treaties are necessary to receive the "help" of the *superior* governance, which not only dictates the meaning of illegality and legality through the externalization of borders in Morocco but also furthers the conceptualization that the irregular and undocumented subjects are always from the Global South; the Western subject cannot be from the European Union or North America precisely because s/he was born in the geopolitical territory.

The Euro-Mediterranean Partnership established an association between the EU and Mediterranean countries. Association agreements with Arab countries increased EU cooperation and financial funding, totaling 3 billion euros annually (Bicchi, 2007). Through this, Brussels, where the partnership was inaugurated, attempted to enhance the EU's influence and increase its soft power in the region under the banner of reinforcing peace in the Middle East (Pace, 2007). The political discourse and actual funding to support MENA countries meant that Europe was trying to make these countries "European," a neocolonial trope that fails to address key issues such as immigration, kleptocracy, and infrastructure gaps (Zaiotti, 2007). Instead, it continues to reinforce the idea that Europe is better than these countries and will never reach the standards it has set, which fuels their need to engage in the neoliberal debt-and-loan cycle (Amin, 2009). Hence, the dismissal and negligence through which the drowned bodies are treated in the Mediterranean becomes excused since Europe is clearly defining who can or cannot be illegal through its securitization (Albahari, 2015). In the neoliberal formulation, the "illegal" is to be blamed because not only is Europe helping them, but Europe also externalizes its borders to stop the phenomenon (Vaughan-Williams, 2015).

However, the externalization of borders is already perceived as a competent and thorough process to guarantee the safety and legality of migrants. Yet, this assumption evades the actual incompetence at the borders. That is, even when irregular migrants are intercepted, they move to cities and areas that are still close to the borders and repeat the process because the discourse of the European Heaven continues. I would further argue that the would-be migrant's expectations and aspirations to migrate "illegally" are not based solely on employment but on the socio-political-economic necessity for the subject to be considered a person rather than a subjugated living thing. The failure of governance and the overt centralization of power in the Moroccan state continue to legitimize the discourse that Moroccans cannot be considered persons if they remain in Morocco. Leaving and the symbolic ramifications of what the youth call "Harba" (which could be translated to running away hurriedly) is exactly running away from the death world, not because it does not provide opportunity, but also and dominantly because the subject feels as a living thing, without rights or right to rights. Everyday discourse through Movies (Bahmad, 2013), jokes (Sabry, 2005), and even the internet (Benharrousse, 2020) legitimize the need to leave because there is no protection for their rights.

The 2021 Fnideq Crisis proved the state's consideration of its own populace as nothing but political tools and living things to pressure Spain politically. The crisis demonstrates the complex intersection of market-driven aspirations and state power. The pre-migratory expectations of Moroccan youth, shaped by neoliberal promises of individuality, self-actualization, and socio-economic agency in Europe, become weaponized tools in international diplomacy. This manipulation of border controls demonstrates an implicit recognition of how specific populations are rendered simultaneously vital to and disposable within state projects. The strategic loosening of borders capitalizes on pre-existing neoliberal subjectivities that position Europe as the socio-economic and infrastructural utopia while simultaneously demonstrating the state's power to manipulate these aspirations for diplomatic leverage.

The differential application of border control, its strategic loosening, and subsequent tightening demonstrates how necropolitical power operates not through absolute prohibition but through calibrated modulation, revealing the sophisticated interplay between neoliberal governmentality and sovereign power, where the state's ability to regulate movement becomes a form of political capital. When Morocco allowed thousands to risk their lives through the irregular crossing, it engaged in a calculated form of political maneuvering, leveraging the perceived gap between local economic precarity and European prosperity. This dynamic illustrates the profound tension between neoliberal ideology's promotion of unfettered capital movement and the reality of highly regulated human mobility. The Moroccan state's actions expose this contradiction by temporarily aligning human mobility with capital mobility, ultimately reinforcing sovereign power rather than individual agency.

The response of European authorities, particularly Spain's deployment of military forces, reveals how contemporary border regimes operate through multilateral exercises of sovereign power. This dynamic illustrates how states balance their exercise of power through the mutual recognition of their capacity to instrumentalize human life. Thus, the crisis exposes how pre-migratory expectations serve as diplomatic leverage within the complex architecture of contemporary border control. This process reveals the profound imbrication of neoliberal subjectivity with necropolitical governance in contemporary border regimes, where human mobility becomes both the subject and instrument of international power relations. The pre-existing desires and aspirations of Moroccan youth, shaped by decades of neoliberal discourse promoting access to the free market, entrepreneurship, wealth, and socio-economic agency, become weaponized within diplomatic negotiations. The temporal suspension of border control reveals how contemporary sovereignty operates through the power to exclude and the strategic management of inclusion.

The state is using the dispositif of the person through neoliberalism. It is already comprehensive of the discourse around the binarism between Morocco as a death world and Europe as salvation from socio-economic fixity and personhood negation. Still, the subject's recognition as a person is contingent upon their ability to maximize their biopolitical power (Foucault, 2008) within the capitalist market. This means that individuals are only considered valuable and worthy of recognition when they conform to idealized performances dictated by market forces (Ong, 2006). In this paradigm, actual living beings are constantly pressured to meet these expectations, and failure to do so results in their relegation to the status of disposable things (Butler, 2004). The neoliberal subject, imbued with the illusion of complete responsibility for their fate within their community, risks becoming part of a population viewed as expendable (Lemke, 2001). Neoliberalism creates a new paradigm that blurs the boundaries between a person and a natural thing, where the configurations of human existence are intertwined with the neoliberal utopia of universal human rights (Brown, 2015). Within this context, the rights-bearing person is afforded protections and immunities that are denied to other living beings lacking such rights (Douzinas, 2007). Hence, the Western "person" is already considered a person because their currency underpins the world's new order, and their travel is not limited, since travel to the Global South would be cheaper. In this formulation, the "living thing" from the Global South is already situated. It will never be able to maximize its economic biopower on the same scale as the Western "persons."

The status of personhood in neoliberalism presupposes a punishing demand for constant economic biopower maximization. This creates a precarious state in which an increasing number of subjects are deemed ineligible for personhood (Standing, 2011). The question of precarity becomes already embedded in one's mind. Even those who qualify as persons within this framework are only temporarily immune to being reduced to the status of living things, as they are constantly threatened with losing their privileged position. Hence, for immigrants, market participation intensifies rather than ameliorates immigrant vulnerability within the neoliberal structuring structure (Benharrousse, 2025). One can even further argue that the status of bare life is always intertwined with the neoliberal dispositif, especially since personhood is not fixed but is constantly in flux (Agamben, 1998). It is important to note that significant wealth can provide a degree of insulation from being categorized as a mere living thing in neoliberal societies. Those who possess substantial wealth are often shielded from the dehumanizing effects of market forces and are more likely to maintain their status as recognized persons (Sassen, 2016). Even wealth accumulation does not guarantee immunity from the volatility and competition inherent in global capitalism (Piketty, 2014).

The precariousness of wealth and the potential for its loss further underline the fragility of neoliberal subjectivity (Harvey, 2007). The neoliberal dispositif perpetuates a dichotomy between persons and living things, positioning the former as idealized and protected while relegating the latter to disposability (Mbembe, 2003). The Fnideq incident grounds the state's treatment of its own "nationals" as disposable because they want to "exit" the country. The neoliberal subject's constant pursuit of maximization not just of wealth but also of personhood creates a perceived precarious state where even those deemed persons are perpetually at risk of being reduced to the status of living things (Lorey, 2015). One's positionality as a Moroccan already puts one in a self-perceived state of being a living thing. This, reinforced through the volatility and competition of global capitalism, means that such privileges are inherently precarious and subject to potential loss (Streeck, 2016). By criminalizing unauthorized entry and creating a complex web of legal statuses, these measures strip migrants of their personhood, reducing them to administrative categories and impersonal corporeal things. Focusing on interception, detention, and expulsion further reinforces the idea that these individuals are not "persons" worthy of rights and protection but rather problems to be managed or eliminated.

The Irregular Migrant as Disposable, not Immunized

The schism between disposability and immunization grounds the would-be and irregular migrant as unworthy of immunization, thereby denying them personhood. Kleptocracy, corruption, and a lack of infrastructure situate Moroccan would-be migrants as already unable to achieve personhood through maximizing their biopolitical power within the capitalist market (Hibou, 2011). Hence, the idea of Europe as a space of opportunity and personhood emerges as the ultimate space in which the person can be deemed worthy of immunization and become part of the community, thereby maximizing one's socio-cultural, political, and economic standing within society (De Genova, 2017). The idea of Europe becomes a discursive structure of binarism between a perceived never-experienced Europe and a lived, over-experienced Morocco, wherein the subject is a living dead if they continue to live in the *death-worlds* with the possibility of salvation through irregularity (Mbembe, 2003; Mbembe, 2019). Accordingly, to achieve personhood, the subject "naturally" must seek Europe to deserve human rights as a citizen of a European country and be worthy of worldwide consideration (Fassin, 2011). The Mediterranean crisis has become an issue in which European countries deliberately neglect irregular migrants drowning near their territories, irrespective of international law and human rights (Cuttitta, 2018). Neglect is epistemic and political against "illegality" and a fundamental caesura of persons and corporeal things. Moreover, inadequate search-and-rescue operations are a critical factor contributing to the high mortality rates in the Mediterranean (Tazzioli, 2016). Despite international legal obligations, several European governments have adopted increasingly restrictive migration policies, reducing search-and-rescue missions (Carrera et al., 2019).

These policies prioritize deterrence and border control over humanitarian considerations, leaving migrants stranded in distressing and life-threatening situations (Andersson, 2014). Instead of taking responsibility, European countries speak of the naturalness of irregular immigrants as if they were seeking "civilization" irregularly (Balibar, 2004). Following the neoliberal argument of migration for employment, it becomes a self-evident argument that the deaths are the living dead's fault. Therefore, the irregular migrant is blamed because they internalized the myth Europe has forwarded through its policies and programs as the optimal space for civilization and democracy (Žižek, 2016). The consideration of irregular migration as a "natural" process by which the subject becomes a person beyond the status of a living thing is perceived as self-evident (Aradau and Tazzioli, 2020). Accordingly, the would-be migrants are to be blamed because their nation-state has failed to provide adequate infrastructure, and because Europe consistently positions itself as a rich, sovereign power capable of transforming the MENA region through actual financial aid and policies reinforcing democracy and personhood (Huysmans, 2006).

To address this humanitarian crisis, it is crucial to go beyond the statistics and recognize the inherent discursive structures and necropolitical formation, which structure Moroccan would-be migrants as living things and Europeans as persons (Vaughan-Williams, 2015). Another discourse that furthers the international belief in would-be migrants' disposability in the Mediterranean migration crisis is the prevailing perception of irregular migrants' bodies as waste (Mbembe, 2003). This dehumanization stems from a toxic combination of factors, including deep-rooted xenophobia, racism, and a perception that irregular migrants pose a threat to the social, economic, and cultural fabric of host countries (De Genova, 2018). As a result, the loss of human life in the Mediterranean is often met with indifference, silence, or even hostility (Cuttitta, 2018) because the irregular migrant is perceived as not a person with protective rights but as a corporeal thing that does not have the right to rights. The disposable is already entrenched in a "waste" discourse that deems these irregulars as unworthy not just of life but of rights. Hence, European countries have insufficient search-and-rescue operations, especially after the 2015 migration crisis (Cusumano, 2019).

Despite the legal obligation to rescue those in distress at sea, several European governments have adopted increasingly restrictive migration policies, leading to a reduction in rescue missions and leaving migrants stranded in treacherous waters (Carrera et al., 2019). The obligation is discharged when the subject is from the Global South, and even more so when they are irregular. The apparent acceptance of these deaths by European authorities, evidenced by inadequate rescue operations and the prioritization of border control over *human* safety, sends a clear message about the value placed on migrant lives from the Global South, furthering the idea that they are not persons. This tacit acceptance of migrant deaths at sea is a stark manifestation of the necropolitical structuring of who is worthy of being immunized. The frequency of these tragedies and their representation in the media contribute to a normalization of migrant disposability in the public consciousness and further reinforcement of the belief in the migrants' corporeal, waste status.

Media Representation as Dehumanization

The construction of Mediterranean migrants as disposable subjects is not solely the result of historical legacies and policy frameworks. Media representation plays a crucial role in shaping public perception and reinforcing the "dispositif of the Person" (Esposito, 2012). The mediation of migration issues significantly influences public discourse and policy responses, often contributing to the dehumanization and othering of migrants (Chouliaraki and Stolic, 2017). News coverage of Mediterranean migration frequently employs a "numbers game" approach, reducing complex human stories to impersonal data and statistics (Vollmer, 2011). This quantification of migration depersonalizes migrants, presenting them as an undifferentiated mass rather than individuals with unique experiences and identities.

The persistent use of terms like "illegal immigrants" or "boat people" in media discourse further contributes to this dehumanization process, stripping migrants of their identities and histories (Howarth and Ibrahim, 2012). Images of overcrowded boats or large groups at borders are frequently employed, contributing to a sense of invasion or crisis (Bleiker et al., 2013). This visual framing reinforces the perception of migrants as a faceless "other" attempting to "ruin" the status quo through informality and "illegality" to justify overt securitization and negligence of migrants at sea. Chouliaraki and Stolic (2017) argue that such imagery, particularly in the context of the "refugee crisis," often oscillates between portraying migrants as victims or threats, rarely allowing for more nuanced representations that recognize their full humanity and agency.

When individual stories are presented in media narratives, they often focus on tragedy or criminality. Horsti (2012) notes that these narratives tend to fall into two main categories: the "victim frame" and the "intruder frame." The victim frame, while potentially eliciting sympathy, still positions migrants as passive subjects lacking agency. The intruder frame, on the other hand, presents migrants as threats to social order and national security. Despite their apparent opposition, both frames contribute to constructing migrants as "others" who do not fully belong in European societies, not persons, which will reinforce informality and unthrowable waste. This media framing interacts with historical prejudices and policy decisions to create a self-reinforcing cycle of migrant disposability and militarization of borders. Public perception shaped by these representations influences policy decisions, providing new material for media coverage and perpetuating the construction of migrants as less-than-human subjects. As Aas and Gundhus (2015) argue, this cycle contributes to the "crimmigration" phenomenon, where immigration control becomes increasingly intertwined with criminal justice, further entrenching the perceived disposability of migrant lives.

Moreover, the selective visibility of migrant experiences in media coverage contributes to what Butler (2009) terms the "differential distribution of grievability." The deaths of migrants at sea, while occasionally sparking temporary outrage, are often presented as inevitable tragedies rather than as consequences of specific policies or societal attitudes. This framing normalizes the loss of migrant lives, reinforcing their status as disposable subjects who are not worthy of immunity precisely because they are not persons but living things. The media's role in constructing migrants as disposable subjects is not monolithic, however. Alternative media narratives and counter-discourses exist, often emerging from activist groups, NGOs, and some journalistic practices that seek to humanize migrants and challenge dominant representations (Georgiou and Zaborowski, 2017). These counter-narratives attempt to reframe the discussion around migration, emphasizing the humanity of migrants and their rights as persons. However, such voices often struggle to compete with mainstream media narratives in shaping broad public perception.

The haunting images of overcrowded boats left adrift, with migrants pleading for help, symbolize the systemic discursive structuring of their lives as disposable and unworthy of human rights (Pezzani and Heller, 2013). The irregular immigrants, because they have no neoliberal biopower nor from "first-world" countries, do not deserve to be saved (Fassin, 2011). Secondly, the criminalization of humanitarian actors and organizations dedicated to saving lives at sea further exemplifies the perception of irregular migrants as disposable (Cusumano and Villa, 2020). By impeding their vital work through legal restrictions, bureaucratic hurdles, and smear campaigns, governments inadvertently contribute to a climate that dismisses the worth of these vulnerable individuals (Fekete, 2018). Humanitarian aid workers, who risk their lives to provide assistance and rescue at sea, face increasing obstacles, making it clear that the bodies of irregular migrants are deemed unworthy of salvation (Stierl, 2018). Moreover, the language employed in political discourse and media coverage also perpetuates the devaluation of irregular migrants' bodies (Andersson, 2014). Terms such as "illegal aliens," "swarms," or "invaders" dehumanize and stigmatize these individuals, reinforcing the notion that their lives are disposable and their suffering inconsequential. Such rhetoric, which finds its way into public consciousness, fuels a hostile environment that erodes empathy and solidarity, further marginalizing irregular migrants and reinforcing their self-perception of waste (Kynsilehto, 2018). Mainstream media often reinforces historical prejudices and supports restrictive policy frameworks through framing choices, visual representations, and narrative structures. This media environment interacts with other factors—including colonialism's historical legacies and the evolution of migration policies—to create and maintain a 'dispositif of the Person' that systematically denies full personhood to Mediterranean migrants.

Conclusion

Throughout this chapter, I have traced how historical legacies, policy frameworks, and media representations work to construct Mediterranean migrants as disposable subjects who are not eligible to be persons. The colonial history and economic disparities between Europe and North Africa set the stage for differentiated perceptions of who is worthy of being a person with the right to rights. These dynamics are reinforced through policies that criminalize migration and prioritize border control over human lives by reducing the migrant to a corporeal "other" without the right to immunity. Media representations further reinforce these perceptions, reducing complex human experiences to impersonal statistics or threatening narratives. Together, these factors create and maintain a "dispositif of the Person" that systematically denies full personhood to Mediterranean migrants, rendering them disposable.

The perilous journeys undertaken by Mediterranean migrants and the frequent tragedies starkly manifest this constructed disposability. The apparent acceptance of migrant deaths at sea by European authorities—evidenced by inadequate rescue operations and the prioritization of border control over human safety—is a clear example of necropolitics in action. The normalization of these tragedies in public consciousness further entrenches the perception of migrant lives as expendable. This complex interplay of historical, political, and social factors creates a system in which the disposability of Mediterranean migrants is accepted and often seen as an inevitable consequence of irregular migration itself. The "dispositif of the Person," as conceptualized by Esposito, operates in this context to systematically exclude certain groups from the category of fully recognized persons deserving of rights and protection. However, it is crucial to realize that this construction of disposability is neither natural nor inevitable. It is a product of specific historical processes, policy decisions, and cultural narratives, all of which can be challenged and changed. Alternative narratives and approaches exist, often emerging from activist groups, NGOs, and critical scholarship. These counter-discourses seek to rehumanize migrants, emphasizing their individual stories, their rights as persons, and the complex factors driving migration.

Moving forward, it is imperative that we critically examine and challenge the processes through which migrant disposability is constructed and maintained. This requires a multifaceted approach that addresses historical inequalities, reforms restrictive policies, and promotes more nuanced and humanizing media representations. By recognizing the full personhood of Mediterranean migrants and challenging the "dispositif of the Person" that renders them disposable, we can work toward more just and humane approaches to migration management. By understanding these processes, we can begin to imagine and work toward alternatives that recognize the inherent dignity and worth of all human lives, regardless of their migration status or origin. This shift in perspective is a moral imperative and a necessary step toward developing more effective and humane responses to the complex challenges of Mediterranean migration in the twenty-first century.

Acknowledgments

An earlier version of this chapter was presented at the International Conference on Immunity and Community, held at Ibn Zohr University in November 2022. I am grateful to the conference participants for their thoughtful engagement and valuable feedback. I wish to express my sincere gratitude to Dr. Jamal Bahmad for his insightful comments, enriching conversations, and critical perspectives, which significantly strengthened this work. I also extend my thanks to the editors for their meticulous attention and dedicated efforts in bringing this volume to fruition. Finally, I am grateful to the editorial and production team at Bloomsbury for their careful copyediting and support throughout the publication process.

References

Aas, Katja Franko, and Helene O. I. Gundhus. "Policing Humanitarian Borderlands: Frontex, Human Rights and the Precariousness of Life." *British Journal of Criminology* 55, no. 1 (2015): 1–18.

Agamben, Giorgio. *Homo Sacer: Sovereign Power and Bare Life*. Stanford: Stanford University Press, 1998.

Albahari, Maurizio. *Crimes of Peace: Mediterranean Migrations at the World's Deadliest Border*. Philadelphia: University of Pennsylvania Press, 2015.

Amin, Samir. *Eurocentrism: Modernity, Religion, and Democracy: A Critique of Eurocentrism and Culturalism*. New York: Monthly Review Press, 2009.

Andersson, Ruben. *Illegality, Inc.: Clandestine Migration and the Business of Bordering Europe*. Oakland: University of California Press, 2014.

Aradau, Claudia, and Martina Tazzioli. "Biopolitics Multiple: Migration, Extraction, Subtraction." *Millennium* 48, no. 2 (2020): 198–220.

Bahmad, Jamal. "From Casablanca to Casanegra: Neoliberal Globalization and Disaffected Youth in Moroccan Urban Cinema." *Middle East Journal of Culture and Communication* 6, no. 1 (2013): 15–35. https://doi.org/10.1163/18739865-00503002.

Balibar, Étienne. *We, the People of Europe? Reflections on Transnational Citizenship*. Princeton: Princeton University Press, 2004.

Benharrousse, Rachid. "Against the Homeland: Popular Exilic Antagonism through 'Azzouz Is Mad.'" *Runas. Journal of Education and Culture* 1, no. 1 (2020): 57–65. https://doi.org/10.46652/runas.v1i1.6.

Benharrousse, Rachid. "The Immigrant as Other: Racial Capitalism, Neoliberalism, and Necropolitics in Laila Lalami's The Other Americans." *Prague Journal of English Studies 14 (2)*, (2025): 173–94. https://doi.org/10.14712/23362685.5085.

Bhambra, Gurminder K. "Postcolonial Reflections on Sociology." *Sociology* 50, no. 5 (2016): 960–966.

Bicchi, Federica. *European Foreign Policy Making Toward the Mediterranean*. New York: Palgrave Macmillan, 2007.

Bigo, Didier. "Security and Immigration: Toward a Critique of the Governmentality of Unease." *Alternatives* 27, no. 1 (2002): 63–92.

Bleiker, Roland, David Campbell, Emma Hutchison, and Xzarina Nicholson. "The Visual Dehumanisation of Refugees." *Australian Journal of Political Science* 48, no. 4 (2013): 398–416.

Boswell, Christina. *European Migration Policies in Flux: Changing Patterns of Inclusion and Exclusion*. Oxford: Blackwell Publishing, 2003.

Brown, Wendy. *Undoing the Demos: Neoliberalism's Stealth Revolution*. New York: Zone Books, 2015.

Brown, Wendy. *Walled States, Waning Sovereignty*. New York: Zone Books, 2018.

Buoli, Alice. "Beyond the Border: Exploring Cross-Scalar Socio-Spatial Dynamics of Conflict, Resistance, and Encounter at the Ceuta–Morocco Borderscapes." *Regional Studies Regional Science* 1, no. 1 (2014): 301–309, https://doi.org10.1080/21681376.2014.977941.

Butler, Judith. *The Force of Nonviolence: An Ethico-Political Bind.* London: Verso, 2019.

Butler, Judith. *Frames of War: When Is Life Grievable?* London: Verso, 2009.

Butler, Judith. *Precarious Life: The Powers of Mourning and Violence*. London: Verso, 2004.

Carling, Jørgen. "Migration Control and Migrant Fatalities at the Spanish-African Borders." *International Migration Review* 41, no. 2 (2007): 316–343, https://doi.org10.1111/j.1747-7379.2007.00070.x.

Carling, Jørgen, and María Hernández-Carretero. "Protecting Europe and Protecting Migrants? Strategies for Managing Unauthorised Migration from Africa." *The British Journal of Politics and International Relations* 13, no. 1 (2011): 42–58.

Carrera, Sergio. "The EU Border Management Strategy: FRONTEX and the Challenges of Irregular Immigration in the Canary Islands." *CEPS Working Document* No. 261, 2007.

Carrera, Sergio, Valsamis Mitsilegas, Jennifer Allsopp, and Lina Vosyliūtė. *Policing Humanitarianism: EU Policies Against Human Smuggling and their Impact on Civil Society*. London: Hart Publishing, 2019.

Cassarino, Jean-Pierre. "Informalising Readmission Agreements in the EU Neighbourhood." *The International Spectator* 42, no. 2 (2007): 179–196.
Cassarino, Jean-Pierre. "Readmission Policy in the European Union." *European Parliament's Committee on Civil Liberties, Justice and Home Affairs*, 2010.
Castles, Stephen. "Understanding Global Migration: A Social Transformation Perspective." *Journal of Ethnic and Migration Studies* 36, no. 10 (2010): 1565–1586.
Chouliaraki, Lilie, and Tijana Stolic. "Rethinking Media Responsibility in the Refugee 'Crisis': A Visual Typology of European News." *Media, Culture & Society* 39, no. 8 (2017): 1162–1177.
Collyer, Michael. "In-Between Places: Trans-Saharan Transit Migrants in Morocco and the Fragmented Journey to Europe." *Antipode* 39, no. 4 (2007): 668–690.
Cusumano, Eugenio. "Migrant Rescue as Organized Hypocrisy: EU Maritime Missions Offshore Libya Between Humanitarianism and Border Control." *Cooperation and Conflict* 54, no. 1 (2019): 3–24.
Cusumano, Eugenio, and Matteo Villa. "From 'Angels' to 'Vice Smugglers': The Criminalization of Sea Rescue NGOs in Italy." *European Journal on Criminal Policy and Research* 26, no. 1 (2020): 97–115.
Cuttitta, Paolo. "Repoliticization Through Search and Rescue? Humanitarian NGOs and Migration Management in the Central Mediterranean." *Geopolitics* 23, no. 3 (2018): 632–660.
De Genova, Nicholas. "The Borders of 'Europe' and the European Question." In *The Borders of "Europe": Autonomy of Migration, Tactics of Bordering*, edited by Nicholas De Genova, 1–35. Durham: Duke University Press, 2017.
De Genova, Nicholas. *The Borders of "Europe": Autonomy of Migration, Tactics of Bordering*. Durham: Duke University Press, 2017.
De Genova, Nicholas. "The 'Migrant Crisis' as Racial Crisis: Do Black Lives Matter in Europe?" *Ethnic and Racial Studies* 41, no. 10 (2018): 1765–1782.
De Genova, Nicholas. "Migrant 'Illegality' and Deportability in Everyday Life." *Annual Review of Anthropology* 31, no. 1 (2002): 419–447.
De Haas, Hein. "The Myth of Invasion: The Inconvenient Realities of African Migration to Europe." *Third World Quarterly* 29, no. 7 (2008): 1305–1322.
Del Sarto, Raffaella A., and Tobias Schumacher. "From EMP to ENP: What's at Stake with the European Neighbourhood Policy towards the Southern Mediterranean?" *European Foreign Affairs Review* 10, no. 1 (2005): 17–38.
Douzinas, Costas. *Human Rights and Empire: The Political Philosophy of Cosmopolitanism*. London: Routledge-Cavendish, 2007.
Düvell, Franck. "Paths into Irregularity: The Legal and Political Construction of Irregular Migration." *European Journal of Migration and Law* 13, no. 3 (2011): 275–295.
Esposito, Roberto. *Immunitas: The Protection and Negation of Life*. Cambridge: Polity Press, 2011.

Esposito, Roberto. *Third Person: Politics of Life and Philosophy of the Impersonal.* Cambridge: Polity Press, 2012.
Fassin, Didier. *Humanitarian Reason: A Moral History of the Present.* Berkeley: University of California Press, 2011.
Fekete, Liz. "Migrants, Borders and the Criminalisation of Solidarity in the EU." *Race & Class* 59, no. 4 (2018): 65–83.
Ferrer-Gallardo, Xavier. "The Spanish-Moroccan Border Complex: Processes of Geopolitical, Functional and Symbolic Rebordering." *Political Geography* 27, no. 3 (2008): 301–321.
Foucault, Michel. *The Birth of Biopolitics: Lectures at the Collège de France, 1978-1979.* Basingstoke: Palgrave Macmillan, 2008.
Geddes, Andrew. "Europe's Border Relationships and International Migration Relations." *JCMS: Journal of Common Market Studies* 43, no. 4 (2005): 787–806.
Georgiou, Myria, and Rafal Zaborowski. "Media Coverage of the 'Refugee Crisis': A Cross-European Perspective." *Council of Europe Report*, 2017.
Gibney, Matthew J. "Asylum and the Expansion of Deportation in the United Kingdom." *Government and Opposition* 43, no. 2 (2008): 146–167.
Gillespie, Richard. "A 'Union for the Mediterranean' . . . or for the EU?" *Mediterranean Politics* 13, no. 2 (2008): 277–286.
Gillespie, Richard. "This Stupid Little Island: A Neighbourhood Confrontation in the Western Mediterranean." *International Politics* 43, no. 1 (2006): 110–132.
Godenau, Dirk. "An Institutional Approach to Bordering in Islands: The Canary Islands on the African-European Migration Routes." *Island Studies Journal* 9, no. 1 (2014): 39–56.
González-Enríquez, Carmen. "Spain, the Cheap Model. Irregularity and Regularisation as Immigration Management Policies." *European Journal of Migration and Law* 11, no. 2 (2009): 139–157.
Harvey, David. *A Brief History of Neoliberalism.* Oxford: Oxford University Press, 2007.
Harvey, David. *The Anti-Capitalist Chronicles.* London: Pluto Press, 2020.
Hernández-Carretero, María, and Jørgen Carling. "Beyond 'Kamikaze Migrants': Risk Taking in West African Boat Migration to Europe." *Human Organization* 71, no. 4 (2012): 407–416.
Hibou, Béatrice. *The Force of Obedience: The Political Economy of Repression in Tunisia.* Cambridge: Polity Press, 2011.
Horsti, Karina. "Humanitarian Discourse Legitimating Migration Control: FRONTEX Public Communication." In *Migrations: Interdisciplinary Perspectives*, edited by Michi Messer, Renee Schroeder, and Ruth Wodak, 297–308. Vienna: Springer, 2012.
Howarth, Anita, and Yasmin Ibrahim. "Threat and Suffering: The Liminal Space of 'The Jungle.'" In *Liminal Landscapes: Travel, Experience and Spaces In-between*, edited by Hazel Andrews and Les Roberts, 200–216. London: Routledge, 2012.

Huysmans, Jef. *The Politics of Insecurity: Fear, Migration and Asylum in the EU*. London: Routledge, 2006.

Ikuteyijo, Lanre Olusegun. "The Impact of European Union Migration Policies on Irregular Migration in Sub-Saharan Africa." In *Migration, Diasporas and Citizenship*, edited by Belachew Gebrewold and Tendayi Bloom, 97–113. London: Palgrave Macmillan, 2014.

IOM (International Organization for Migration). "Missing Migrants Project." 2021. https://missingmigrants.iom.int/.

Khosravi, Shahram. *'Illegal' Traveller: An Auto-Ethnography of Borders*. Basingstoke: Palgrave Macmillan, 2010.

Kynsilehto, Anitta. "Mobilities, Politics, and Solidarities." *Peace Review* 30, no. 3 (2018): 371–378.

Lavenex, Sandra, and Emek M. Uçarer. "The External Dimension of Europeanization: The Case of Immigration Policies." *Cooperation and Conflict* 39, no. 4 (2004): 417–443.

Lemke, Thomas. "The Birth of Bio-Politics: Michel Foucault's Lecture at the Collège de France on Neo-Liberal Governmentality." *Economy and Society* 30, no. 2 (2001): 190–207.

Levinson, Amanda. "Regularization of Unauthorized Migrants: Literature Survey and Country Case Studies." *Centre on Migration, Policy and Society*. University of Oxford, 1994.

Lorey, Isabell. *State of Insecurity: Government of the Precarious*. London: Verso, 2015.

Lutterbeck, Derek. "Policing Migration in the Mediterranean." *Mediterranean Politics* 11, no. 1 (2006): 59–82.

Mbembe, Achille. *Necropolitics*. Durham: Duke University Press, 2019.

Mbembe, Achille. "Necropolitics." *Public Culture* 15, no. 1 (2003): 11–40.

Ong, Aihwa. *Neoliberalism as Exception: Mutations in Citizenship and Sovereignty*. Durham: Duke University Press, 2006.

Pace, Michelle. "The Construction of EU Normative Power." *JCMS: Journal of Common Market Studies* 45, no. 5 (2007): 1041–1064.

Pezzani, Lorenzo, and Charles Heller. "A Disobedient Gaze: Strategic Interventions in the Knowledge(s) of Maritime Borders." *Postcolonial Studies* 16, no. 3 (2013): 289–298.

Piketty, Thomas. *Capital in the Twenty-First Century*. Cambridge, MA: Harvard University Press, 2014.

Pugh, Michael. "Drowning Not Waving: Boat People and Humanitarianism at Sea." *Journal of Refugee Studies* 17, no. 1 (2004): 50–69.

Sabry, Tarik. "Emigration as Popular Culture: The Case of Morocco." *European Journal of Cultural Studies* 8, no. 1 (2005): 5–22. https://doi.org/10.1177/1367549405049489.

Sassen, Saskia. *Expulsions: Brutality and Complexity in the Global Economy*. Cambridge, MA: Harvard University Press, 2016.

Spijkerboer, Thomas. "The Human Costs of Border Control." *European Journal of Migration and Law* 9, no. 1 (2007): 127–139.

Standing, Guy. *The Precariat: The New Dangerous Class*. London: Bloomsbury Academic, 2011.

Stierl, Maurice. "A Sea of Struggle: Activist Border Interventions in the Mediterranean Sea." *Citizenship Studies* 22, no. 5 (2018): 467–484.

Streeck, Wolfgang. *How Will Capitalism End?: Essays on a Failing System*. London: Verso, 2016.

Tazzioli, Martina. "Border Displacements. Challenging the Politics of Rescue Between Mare Nostrum and Triton." *Migration Studies* 4, no. 1 (2016): 1–19.

Triandafyllidou, Anna. "Controlling Migration in Southern Europe (Part 2): Gate-keeping Strategies." *ARI 8/2010*, Real Instituto Elcano, 2010.

Triandafyllidou, Anna, and Maurizio Ambrosini. "Irregular Immigration Control in Italy and Greece: Strong Fencing and Weak Gate-keeping Serving the Labour Market." *European Journal of Migration and Law* 13, no. 3 (2011): 251–273.

Vaughan-Williams, Nick. *Europe's Border Crisis: Biopolitical Security and Beyond*. Oxford: Oxford University Press, 2015.

Vollmer, Bastian A. "Policy Discourses on Irregular Migration in the EU—'Number Games' and 'Political Games.'" *European Journal of Migration and Law* 13, no. 3 (2011): 317–339.

Weiss, Thomas G. *Humanitarian Challenges and Intervention*. New York: Routledge, 2018.

Zaiotti, Ruben. "Of Friends and Fences: Europe's Neighbourhood Policy and the 'Gated Community Syndrome.'" *Journal of European Integration* 29, no. 2 (2007): 143–162.

Žižek, Slavoj. *Against the Double Blackmail: Refugees, Terror and Other Troubles with the Neighbours*. London: Allen Lane, 2016.

5

Pandemics and Socio-Economic Reforms

A Comparative-Historical Perspective on Infectious Diseases' Impact on Societies

Sara Tabza and Mohamed Belamghari

Throughout the course of history, infectious diseases have had an impact on societies causing suffering and loss of life. They have also brought to light the vulnerabilities in our healthcare systems, public health measures, social policies, and cultural norms. In addition to the devastating effects on lives, these pandemics have led to changes in how we approach our surroundings and how we interact with one another. As a result, societies have been forced to reassess and restructure different aspects including governance, public healthcare systems, measures, and social policies. The Black Death is one of the most important reminders of the abysmal impact that pandemics can have on society. The devastation it brought upon medieval Europe has been extensively documented, and its consequences were far-reaching. According to Piret and Boivin (2021), the Black Death catalyzed significant social reforms, forcing communities to reevaluate public health measures. This resulted in the implementation of stricter quarantine protocols, improved sanitation standards, and the establishment of hospitals and other vital healthcare infrastructure that were much needed in later epochs of similar pandemics. Moreover, the labor shortages caused by the Black Death had unexpected positive effects.

Similarly, the Spanish Flu pandemic of 1918–19 had a lasting impact on societies around the globe. Its destructive reach highlighted the necessity for robust public health systems. As Matsumoto et al. (2021) point out, this crisis catalyzed the establishment of comprehensive measures to prevent and control diseases. This included the formation of national health agencies, the implementation of efficient disease surveillance and reporting mechanisms, and significant progress in the development and distribution of vaccines.

Despite the significant death toll caused by cholera, the outbreak led to major economic and infrastructural reforms in urban areas. The recurrences of cholera in the nineteenth century, especially in Paris and Hamburg, highlighted the ineffectiveness of the old city sanitation and brought about the necessity for a civilized urban infrastructure. The enhanced sewerage systems and effective water supply ensured the well-being of the population in urban environments and lowered the rate of mortality (Plößl & Just, 2022). Additionally, and due to the improved urban layout of European cities and reduction of mortality rates, cholera also contributed to economic growth by attracting businesses.

One does not have to look far back in history for examples of social reforms brought about by pandemics. Covid-19 has proven itself comparable to historical crises such as the Plague, the Spanish Flu, or cholera in shaping society's norms. In fact, it has also acted as a catalyst for the widespread adoption of digital transformation worldwide. Recognizing the need for safety, governments and institutions swiftly embraced digital tools, enabling remote work, online education, telehealth, and contactless transactions. While primarily aimed at curbing the spread of the virus, these measures have also sparked a profound transformation toward a more digitalized future, impacting critical areas like education, healthcare, and business.

Though this chapter mostly highlights the positive impacts of pandemics on societies, it is noteworthy to acknowledge that pandemics have highlighted the disparities, injustices, vulnerabilities, and unequal distribution of opportunities within societies as well. Pandemics not only inspire the need for reassessment and improvements in healthcare and labor policies, but they can also accentuate pre-existing issues and trigger chaos, profiteering, avarice, and all kinds of hysteria (Thompson, 1921).

To unravel the intricate relationship between infectious diseases and consequent social advancements, we will utilize a comprehensive comparative-historical approach which involves a thorough investigation of past events spanning various time periods and regions. This will enable us to uncover common trends, cause-and-effect relationships, and profound societal shifts brought about by pandemics.

Social and Religious Reforms: The Impact of the Black Death on Medieval Society

The Black Death, a devastating pandemic, swept across Europe in the fourteenth century and is estimated to have wiped out one-third of Europe's population, leading to significant social and economic disruption. This deadly disease spread rapidly, transmitted through fleas or rats and through human contact (Thalassinou et al., 2015). The impact of the Plague on medieval Europe was great, and it led to various reform movements. To understand the depth of the reform triggered by the Black Death, it is vital to understand the social structure of medieval Europe pre-plague first.

The pre-plague medieval Europe was characterized by a hierarchical social structure and a rigid class system. During the medieval period, a hierarchical system known as feudalism reigned supreme. Under this system, land belonged to the nobility and was worked by the lower-class servants known as serfs. The wealthy and powerful lords controlled much of the resources and held significant influence, while the common people, including peasants and serfs, were often impoverished and had limited freedoms (McMichael, 2010). Education and literacy were primarily reserved for the clergy and the nobility, with only a small percentage of the population having access to formal schooling. The church was powerful and provided spiritual guidance and a sense of community. Pre-plague medieval Europe was a fertile ground for social and cultural transformation. The feudal system was already facing challenges before the outbreak of the Black Death. The decline of the Roman Empire and the invasions by barbarian tribes weakened the centralized authority of monarchs, leading to a fragmented society with powerful local lords and landowners (Messager et al., 2022). During this period, life was unbearable for much of the population. People lived in overcrowded villages, relying on subsistence farming for survival and barely survived.

As the population dwindled due to the outbreak of the disease, a shortage of labor emerged, granting the peasants greater autonomy and leverage (Routt, 2004). The lords and nobles, whose estates and control depended on their vassals' forced labor and services, were no longer able to sustain their positions. This presented an opening for the peasants to assert their rights and demand fair treatment. This alteration hastened the demise of the feudal system, causing the traditional social structure to crumble. A notable instance of this can be identified in the Peasants' Revolt of 1381 in England. The primary catalyst for the uprising was the heavy taxation brought about by the Hundred Years' War (Thompson, 1921). However, this reason was merely the final straw for the people because "the socioeconomic changes already driven by other causes would have occurred anyway, merely more slowly, had the plague never struck Europe" (Routt, 2004). The socioeconomic inequalities had become too much to bear, and the acceptance of serfdom had greatly diminished in the wake of the pandemic. Survivors have appropriate possessions and riches that they have never imagined owning. This sudden change of fate, though contributed to the fall of the feudal system, was a double-edged sword. The negative effects will be discussed in the last part of this chapter.

The epoch was characterized by undeniable ramifications of society and the reshuffling of the class hierarchy made it possible for the new rich to set new standards. Though it could be argued whether or not the feudal system brought an advantage to English society, the new condition of luxury that the peasants enjoyed fairly made them richer but definitely made Europe poorer (Thompson, 1921). This is due to the cessation of production for several months, which forced Europe to later seek riches elsewhere. Surprisingly enough, the Black Death may have marked the beginning of European expansion[1] and the exploitation of foreign land because the post-pandemic era gave rise to a "new European political economy [that] became "man-powering": getting other people to work or fight for you by hook or by crook" (Belich, 2016).

Besides the economic and political landscapes, religion was also put into question because of the pandemic. Though the corruption of the church during the medieval period should have easily been the only reason for people to apostatize when the Plague provided an escape (Zentner, 2015), it can't be denied that the search for meaning amid chaos fueled religiosity. The devastating mortality rate brought forth a sense of fear and despair among the people, resulting in a deep introspection of their beliefs. In the face of such widespread death and suffering, some people turned to their faith for solace and answers while others started to question the very idea of religion. This led to a resurgence of different new religious practices and a renewed emphasis on piety and devotion. Monastic orders, in particular, experienced a revival as individuals sought refuge and meaning in their cloistered communities. Monks and nuns dedicated themselves to a life of prayer and contemplation, providing spiritual guidance and support to those struggling to make sense of societal norms and values, leading to increased movements for social reform. One such movement was the rise of charitable organizations and institutions. With so many individuals affected by the Black Death, the need for support and assistance became evident. As a result, charitable organizations, such as hospitals and almshouses, were established to provide aid and care for the sick and destitute.

The other facet of the coin was challenging the church. "People were able to see the 'human' side of the Church that was unable to save them from the onslaught of the plague" (Zentner, 2015, p. 51). Just like the fall of feudalism, the bureaucracy imposed by the Catholic Church due to its focus on worldly materials and political power weakened not only its state but even the devotion of the flock. It is important to note that most Europeans still believed in God but were no longer confident about the ability of the church as an institution (Zentner, 2015).

The pandemic triggered a surge in religious fervor, giving rise to various dissident religious groups that advocated for different versions of Christianity, such as the flagellant movement and the anti-Semitic movement. Followers of the flagellant movement believed that publicly flagellating themselves could serve as a form of penance for not only their sins but also those of others. Unlike the flagellants that sought penance by inflicting punishment upon themselves, other Christians blamed the Jews for the wrath of God upon their people and felt the need to purge their communities by slaughtering Jewish people (Zentner, 2015). Of course, the Plague did not create the tense relationship between Christians and Jews, it only exacerbated it. This was a result of generations of repressed simmering hate toward the Jews, which the church could no longer stop no matter how much it opposed it. Christians at that time questioned the church's aptness to lead the way toward salvation, and they decided to take the matter into their own hands. These movements and more contributed to the fall of the church and the rise of collective action.

The Spanish Flu Pandemic and the Modern Public Health Systems

Another pandemic that swept the world by storm was the Spanish Flu of 1918. Though the name given to this pandemic suggests that this outbreak started in Spain, it did not. The mere reason why it is called the Spanish Flu is because during the First World War Spain was neutral and the press was not censored to report death cases. For other countries involved in the war, spreading information about their ailing soldiers would benefit their enemies (Sowards, 2018). This secrecy about the spread of the virus kept the general public in the dark and exacerbated the situation. In addition to the secrecy, and since the Spanish Flu is a classic crowd respiratory disease that is highly contagious, the abysmal conditions of the military camps and cities of high densities expedited the spread of the pandemic (Spinney, 2020).

The high death toll was very alarming in the new "mass society" era and changes needed to be made urgently. Though vaccines had already been introduced in the late eighteenth century by the English physician Edward Jenner, viruses were "still a little-known branch of the germ family" (Thomes, 2010, p. 50). They were way too small, not as recognizable as bacteria, and pretty difficult to isolate. This made health experts resort to rudimentary transfusion of blood (directly from cured people to sick ones) and several preventive measures such as quarantine and sanitary policing (Wallace, 2020). None of these measures prevented the second and third waves from being so damaging and everything that had been done "proved to be a weak reed to lean upon" (Soper qtd. in Thomes, 2010, p. 51).

According to the CDC[2] and the WHO,[3] the failure to contain the Spanish Flu has directly triggered improvements in different areas such as sanitation practices, healthcare infrastructure, disease surveillance systems, vaccine development and distribution, quarantine measures, labor conditions, and wages of healthcare providers. None of this happened overnight, and the influence of the Spanish Flu is still perceptible in the medical innovations of the century that followed.

In an article titled "'Destroyer and Teacher': Managing the Masses During the 1918–1919 Influenza Pandemic" (2010), Nancy Thomes revisits the lessons learned from the pandemic and explores how it created "new awareness of the problems of disease prevention in a mass society" (p. 49). Thomes speaks of how something as simple as using a handkerchief was considered a triumph. Once health officials had a clear understanding of how the disease spreads through mouth and nose secretions and diluted germs in the air, they attempted to control the spread by drawing "on the strong hygienic program popularized by the anti-TB movement at the turn of the century" (Thomes, 2010, p. 50). In the United States, for example, the National Tuberculosis Association made use of the entertainment industry to raise awareness about the importance of protection against respiratory diseases. Practices such as careful coughing, sneezing, and good hygiene were promoted widely.

The use of gauze masks was a good solution for the threat of droplets in the air, but these masks were mostly used in hospitals and were unavailable to the public. "Women volunteers already accustomed to rolling bandages and knitting socks for the soldiers added making gauze masks to their lists of good deeds" (Thomes,2010, p. 56). In addition to this, handkerchiefs were becoming as popular as the gauze masks. One reason for this is the availability of handkerchiefs and their low price. Authorities advised the people to use hankies when sneezing or coughing and even utilized coercive authorities to ensure compliance (Thomes,2010, p. 57). Stronger enforcement of hygienic laws occurred gradually because lack of personal cleanliness harmed public health, and authorities needed such sanitary regulations to combat the disease. Examples of this were seen in New York where "14 men were reported by sanitary inspectors for using dirty glasses" in a public establishment (Thomes,2010, p. 55). Other examples are anti-spitting laws and bans on public gatherings.

Besides hygiene measures that are still relevant to this day, the Spanish Flu shaped modern medicine, especially epidemiology. This branch of medical science diagnoses disease patterns, causes, and consequences within communities in order to learn how to cope with and avoid future outbreaks. During the 1918–19 pandemic, the concept of virus was unknown, and flu cases were not documented or reported. Thanks to epidemiology, such occurrences are now somewhat anticipated. Further, and as a direct result of the pandemic, health ministries were established in different first world countries, but they were "either left out of cabinet meetings entirely or reduced to pleading for funds" (Spinney, 2020). This was not enough to maintain stability nor control future outbreaks. Additionally, many "countries also recognized the need to coordinate public health at the international level, since clearly, contagious diseases did not respect borders" (Spinney, 2020). This coordination led to what is now called the World Health Organization (WHO), which offers insights and recommendations to respond to health threats on the global scale.

All these post-pandemic changes paved the way for socialized medicine and healthcare as a basic right for citizens around the world (or at least in the first world then). For example, in response to this, countries such as the United Kingdom, which were influenced by the Beveridge Report of 1942, brought about national healthcare systems that were funded by taxation, such as the National Health Service (NHS) which was introduced in 1948. These systems were adopted to ensure that access to healthcare was provided to everyone, regardless of their socioeconomic status. Public healthcare systems were put in place first by Russia and followed by other European countries and the United States. Though this sounds idyllic, it should be noted that the rise of socialized medicine was based on insurance schemes both in Europe and The United States (Spinney, 2020).

Economic Reforms and Pandemics: How Cholera Shaped Urban Infrastructure in the Nineteenth Century

It is somewhat inhuman to consider the silver lining in a devastating catastrophe as that of a pandemic, but one cannot deny the immense positive impact they had on the world. This is relevant to the nineteenth century cholera pandemic as well, which paved the way for massive economic and infrastructural reforms. The first cholera outbreak that took place between 1817 and 1824 started in the Ganges Delta of colonized India, where the cholera bacterium spread through water sources. The disease spread quickly through the British colonial trading networks within Southeast Asia, West Asia, and parts of East Africa. This first wave of cholera signified the advent of the disease on a global scale, but it was mostly confined to the Indian Ocean, with only small forays into Europe.

In the subsequent months several more cholera epidemics occurred in the nineteenth century with each successive wave spreading the disease to the larger section of the world. The second cholera pandemic (1829–51) started to affect Europe and the Americas leading to major outbreaks in cities such as London and Paris that finally figured out that poor hygiene and contaminated water were the reasons behind the spread of the disease[4]. The third pandemic, which began in 1852, had spread far and wide, becoming the deadliest and also creating social advances. An example of this is the the application of mapping by Dr. Snow in identifying the means by which cholera spreads in London in 1854. In 1883, during the Fifth Pandemic, Robert Koch identified Vibrio cholerae, and this new knowledge, along with initiatives to expand modern sanitation systems, led to the modern health systems that slowed down the subsequent pandemics.

The need to curb the fatal disease led to the development of water and sanitation systems and even urban layout. As a result, the improvements in urban infrastructure reduced the mortality rates and improved public health in general. To fathom the magnitude of urbanism in the post-cholera era and the drastic economic and infrastructural shifts, it is important to analyze the pre-pandemic structures that were utterly inadequate.

"Cities enable economies of scale" (Plößl & Just, 2022). They offer administrative and cultural services and quasi-secure living spaces. They also facilitate large-scale production and consumption, which in turn provides labor and capital.[5] Every commercial or cultural exchange, connection, and networking in urban communities benefits the economy as a whole. However, inadequate sanitation infrastructure might lead to economic collapse during a pandemic. This was a tough lesson for Europe during the cholera pandemic. Paris,[6] for example, experienced enormous growth during the nineteenth century as a result of the massive changes brought about by the Industrial Revolution. This, however, was a double-edged sword that magnified the socioeconomic disparities. The population of Paris doubled to over 1 million residents (Kherlakian, 2016) and the higher classes enjoyed clean living environments and health care while the lower classes suffered in the unhygienic living conditions.

In *Paris: The Biography of a City* (2004), Colin Jones details the living conditions and public health issues in Paris amid the rapid growth of the population. Poor people were cramped in poorly constructed neighborhoods with inadequate sewage systems. Waste accumulated in the streets because of the open sewers that were too narrow. Additionally, the water supply was limited for the lower class. Many poor residents did not have access to clean and potable water. Parisians relied on water carriers, fountains, and the Seine River, which were contaminated by waste. Further, the lack of basic medical knowledge fanned the flames; people did not understand the processes by which diseases spread, especially a new one such as the cholera.

Paris was infamous for its unsanitary conditions, and the dire state led to what was known as the Great Stink of 1858, when smell from the raw sewage and waste accumulated became almost intolerable. This event was exacerbated by cholera outbreaks and left the local authorities with no choice but to address the issues of sanitation and public health in the city, which led them to reconsider the state of the sewage systems and to speed up the process of the overall reformation of urban areas. This was expedited "by the citizens demand of change; a demand that signified a new direction in Paris for improved waste control as well as protection of health for its people—a request from a city that largely failed to concern itself with the well-being of its poor residents" (Barnes, 2006).

The modernization of Paris was initiated by Napoleon III, Napoleon Bonaparte's nephew, who ruled France first as its president (1848–52) and then as emperor (1852–70). It is important to note that Napoleon III's ideas of embellishing Paris are founded on two factors. His appreciation of the wide streets of London and beautiful parks during his exile with his family (1830–48) and his willingness to quash any potential rebellion[7] in the well-narrowed streets that barely provided space for barricades in the name of order (Kherlakian, 2016).

In December 1850, Napoleon III announced his intention to renovate Paris. He declared, "Paris is the heart of France. Let us apply our efforts to embellishing this great city. Let us open new streets, make the working-class quarters, which lack air and light, healthier, and let the beneficial sunlight reach everywhere within our walls" (Kherlakian, 2016). When he became emperor, he gained the means to implement his vision with the help of Georges-Eugène Haussmann, whom he appointed as director of public works for the Paris region. Interestingly, Haussmann had no prior training as an architect or urban designer, but he was an astute, capable public administrator (Kherlakian, 2016).

David P. Jordan enumerates Haussmann's genius embellishment of Paris in his 1995 *Transforming Paris: The Life and Labors of Baron Haussmann*. Through his efforts, Haussmann successfully and radically remodeled Paris on a broad scale. His plan was to clear the overcrowded medieval quarters to pave way for spacious tree-planted avenues, new parks, public places, and modern facilities, for instance better sewerage system and gas lighting. This not only beautified the city of Paris but also corrected some of the social ills which affected the residents of that city in terms of health. Some of the changes to the structure of the city included the creation of broad avenues for military use to counter the construction of barricades during uprisings while at the same time making the city more accessible and livelier. Despite a certain number of drawbacks associated with the displacement of people and the high cost of the project, Haussmann made significant contributions to the creation of the modern city of Paris, which earned the title "City of Light," as well as contributing to the further development of other cities worldwide. This, in turn, led to a healthier generation that translated into better output and economic growth of the country.

Similarly, and in other parts of the world, the mid of the nineteenth century was a time of a migration surge to cities. The advancement of better sewage systems was in line with dealing with waste from populated regions. For instance, in the mid-nineteenth century in London, the extensive sewer system designed by Joseph Bazalgette helped to greatly diminish the occurrences of cholera after he directed the waste away from the main source of water supply known as the River Thames (Halliday, 2001). The final important innovation was the source of clean and healthy water supply services. Large cities such as New York embarked on construction of aqueducts like the Croton Aqueduct (1842) for the purpose of conveying water from distant reservoirs to minimize contact with human and animal waste, thus reducing spread of diseases associated with contaminated drinking water (Tarr, 1984). As the municipal districts were growing, these innovations in sanitary engineering proved to be essential in making cities healthier and more sustainable.

The fact that people hardly got sick from waterborne diseases meant that the population grew, and many were available for work and business consumption. Fewer hours were lost because of sickness and health expenses, so the working force increased productivity, affecting industrial and commercial growth of the city. These innovations not only solved very acute problems in providing the population with clean water and improving sewage systems but also contributed significantly to social and economic growth as it created much more favorable conditions for the city's development for both resident population and businessmen (Halliday, 2001). It was such infrastructure developments that contributed to the creation of a healthier urban environment necessary for economic development and productivity, and relieved the economic pressure caused by healthcare costs, proving that there is a link between sanitary advancements and economic performance.

Besides sanitation and infrastructure developments, cholera outbreaks brought about the conception of social amenities such as parks that are open to the public with the aim of enhancing air quality in urban areas. New building codes that focused on limiting the number of occupants of a structure and improving the flow of fresh air to mitigate the effects of poorly designed houses. These changes[8] also prompted the concept of centralized urban management, enabling organized efforts to handle public ailments and the progressive alteration of urban layout to favorability, cleanliness, and health.

The Digital Transformation: Lessons from the Covid-19 Pandemic

Drawing parallels with the previously mentioned pandemics, one cannot deny the significant impact of Covid-19 on our modern world. The Covid-19 pandemic is viewed as the "great accelerator" of digital transformation as it has supported the introduction of various innovative digital technologies in different organizations, accelerating changes in work patterns and business strategies worldwide (Amankwah-Amoah, et al. 2021). To address these measures and stay afloat, businesses turned to these technologies, including cloud computing enabling remote working, video conferencing for meetings, and e-commerce for online shopping. Besides the shift toward paperless systems, these emerging trends have been adopted to enhance competitiveness.

The Covid-19 pandemic brought about a swift transformation in digital retail because of various factors. Firstly, the online shopping trend started due to an increase in lockdowns and social distancing as people began to dislike inconvenience in person. This had a huge impact on e-commerce in different sectors—retail, services, and so on—as businesses started to embrace online sales platforms to satisfy the desire for such sales channels. Furthermore, high-street stores also adopted online platforms to stay afloat during lockdowns. This shift to digitalization created a surge in contactless payment options which in turn increased the popularity of digital wallets, mobile payments, and cashless alternatives.

Besides the digitalization of economic activity, the emergence of Covid-19 has led to changes in the healthcare system; a paradigm shift from Direct Personal Contact (DPC) care to digital care. In 2020, many digital health solutions[9] were quickly implemented to cover issues like patient assessment, monitoring, and communication, especially as such contacts were minimized. Telemedicine also became pivotal for making remote consultations possible through the use of mobile applications and wearables for symptoms tracing and for real-time monitoring of vital signs. In addition, the use of digital platforms meant that the sharing of health data among the various care teams was enhanced and well-coordinated. Together, these solutions ensured patients' care was continued without the risks related to in-person appointments (Gunasekeran et al. 2021).

The use of telehealth in long-term care (LTC) facilities during the Covid-19 pandemic is both beneficial and challenging. Telehealth is a useful utility that ensures delivery services as an essential means of minimizing contacts with patients during periods like lockdowns, for instance. However, senior patients who lack the ability to operate gadgets, navigate the internet, or struggle with their hearing or eyesight still needed more face-to-face consultations (Dai, 2023). Additionally, physicians and healthcare workers believe that telehealth has a positive impact in that patients have better access and improved care, although they also report negative aspects like increased load on LTC staff and technological challenges with limited access to technology, especially in rural areas (Dai, 2023).

In a study titled "Telehealth in Long-term Care Facilities during the Covid-19 Pandemic—Lessons Learned from Patients, Physicians, Nurses, and Healthcare Workers" (2023), the author posits that telehealth will continue to be incorporated into daily LTC care delivery in the post-Covid-19 period because of its relative flexibility and the possibility of enhancing the quality of patient care. However, the author also points out the emphasis on an extra bolster for LTC facilities in rural and other hard-to-reach places due to digital divides. This ranges from investing in technology to supporting telehealth to making certain that healthcare workers are ready to deliver the services, and making sure that the use of telehealth does not eliminate the innate face-to-face interaction by patients with their physicians for a number of ailments that may need contact.

The Covid-19 pandemic also spurred a global movement toward remote jobs by facilitating online technologies usage and changing mindsets about workplace flexibility. In the wake of lockdowns and social distancing norms, companies hurried to put in place remote work arrangements that relied on video conferencing and collaboration platforms. This transition demonstrated the practicality and advantages of mobile working such as higher output, reduced commuting, and better work-life balance. By the same token, firms became aware of the possibility of reducing expenses on office space and overhead issues. This has ushered in a new era of remote work that many organizations rely on as a long-term or permanent option, allowing employees greater flexibility and the chance for companies to tap into talent pools regardless of distance or boundaries. In addition, the pandemic resulted in the advancement of remote work practices, including virtual team-building activities and robust cybersecurity measures, hence improving the experience of working remotely in the present world.

Pandemics and Societal Inequalities: Fear and Divisions

Though pandemics brought so much good to the world and the progress they inspire in different areas of society is profound, it should be noted that they undeniably do exacerbate inequalities, highlight pre-existing issues, and expose loopholes in the social structure. Aside from the "economic chaos, social unrest, high prices, depravation of morals, social and religious hysteria" (Thompson,1921, p. 565), and many other negative consequences caused by the pandemic, there are also some negative effects that boost corruption. An example of this is the high surge in profiteering that comes with such cases of chaos. During the Black Death era, and due to the high death toll, that created vacancies in different state jobs, "thousands of ignorant, incompetent, dishonest men were hastily thrust into public offices" (p. 569). This plunged European societies into maladministration and power abuse all over again. The new appointees were mostly corrupt job seekers with selfish motives that favored their own gain over the benefit of their communities. Of course, one cannot claim that all new appointees were corrupt, but "golden opportunities were afforded to the amateur preacher, the amateur reformer, the pseudo-scientist" and fates of countries were decided by incompetent statesmen (p. 571).

Another negative effect of the Plague on European societies is the decay of civility and manners. The new noblesse or "the nouveau riches" became so overnight and "with the passing of aristocracy passed also the chivalry and courtesy that had distinguished it" (Thompson,1921, p. 568–569). Good manners and civility were replaced by bad manners, flamboyance, and impertinence. Experts in medieval society highlight this change in both literature and historical documents (Thompson,1921). Even decent language died with the old noblesse and obscenity prevailed. Fashion and good taste were also affected by the Black Death. Flamboyant nouveaux riches wanted to flaunt their wealth by excessively wearing jewelry and costumes. This benefited the dressmakers and jewelers, but it was vulgar to say the least (Thompson,1921).

The anti-Semitic movement, mentioned earlier, that rose during the Black Death is one example of the injustices highlighted during pandemics. Though Christians and Jews had their differences, they maintained distance. The chaos and hysteria caused by the pandemic triggered hostility that the church had been opposing for so long. Terror Management Theory suggests explanations of this behavior and further details can be found in Jeff Greenberg, Sheldon Solomon, and Tom Pyszczynski's *The Worm at The Core* (2015) in which the authors explain how individuals respond when reminded of their mortality. In the book, the authors posit that we are haunted by mortality and that the burden of anxiety and the knowledge we live with is both destructive and beneficial at so many levels. We are relentlessly trying to conquer insignificance and redefine the problem of finitude by pondering "our present circumstances in the light of future possibilities to modify our behavior accordingly" (Solomon 2003). It may be noted, without straying too much from our primary purpose, that one of the hypotheses suggested in the previously mentioned book termed Mortality Salience hypothesis suggests that when people are reminded of their mortality, their motivation to sustain and defend their cultural worldviews increases. The threat of annihilation pushes people to pursue their "protective psychological structures" in order to reduce existential anxiety. This motivation can either be productive or destructive; it all depends on the level of adherence to the cultural worldviews one upholds. This theory explains the chaos, hysteria, and hostility between people adhering to different sects of a religion or different religions.

Needless to go far back in history to learn about the different vulnerabilities and unequal distribution of opportunities within societies that are accentuated by pandemics. During the Covid-19 crisis, we witnessed an unprecedented state of emergency, with nations throughout the world implementing lockdown measures. The lockdown may have helped to restrict the spread of the disease, but it also forced many people out of work. People who struggled to maintain themselves or their families were unable to do so under the new emergency legislation. The class disparity grew much greater. Additionally, the media's rhetoric and coverage showed a rise in racism. Bigotry and discrimination against Chinese people were at its peak at the beginning of the Covid-19 crisis just like it did against Africans during the HIV outbreak.

Pandemics have had tremendous effects on nations throughout history; as the physician George Price observed in 1918, they are both "destroyers and teachers" (Price qtd in Tomes, 2010, p. 49). They alter social policies as well as cultural values. Despite the great loss they inflict, pandemics bring about positive consequences. They compel societies to rebuild themselves from their ashes. They have inspired and caused the implementation of much-needed protocols, improved sanitation standards, and the establishment of hospitals and other vital healthcare infrastructure that were much needed in later epochs. They have contributed to the fall of tyrannical institutions and the emergence of better governance. Further, they highlight injustices and inequalities that are sometimes obscured by political correctness. And while it may appear to be a great thing since it must be identified and handled, the negative ramifications are just as destructive as the sickness itself. For further research, this chapter might be extended to a more comprehensible paper that covers more reforms in other aspects of society and more pandemics throughout history.

Notes

1 Check *The World the Plague Made: The Black Death and the Rise of Europe*—July 19, 2022, by James Belich. This book is a panoramic history of how the bubonic plague revolutionized labor, trade, and technology and set the stage for Europe's global expansion.
2 CDC—"Pandemic Influenza: A Guide for the Public."
3 WHO—"A History of Influenza" (archival record).
4 "The Ghost Map: The Story of London's Most Terrifying Epidemic—and How It Changed Science, Cities, and the Modern World" 2007 by Steven Johnson.
5 Check *European Cities After Covid-19* "Urban Function" for more information on the advantages of urban infrastructures on the economy.
6 Please check *Cholera: The Biography* a book by Christopher Hamlin. The book is part of the Biographies of Disease collection.
7 Harvey, David. "The Political Economy of Public Space." *The Politics of Public Space*, eds. Low, Setha and Neil Smith. 2005.
8 Check *Cholera, Urbanization, and the Modern City in The New Urban History and Public Health* by Michael Haines.
9 Check "Digital health during COVID-19: lessons from operationalising new models of care in ophthalmology" (2021). The chapter discusses how digital health solutions such as telehealth, AI decision assistance, and home monitoring have been integrated into ophthalmology care paradigms.

References

Amankwah-Amoah, Joseph et al. "Covid-19 and Digitalization: The Great Acceleration." *Journal of Business Research* 136 (Nov. 2021): 602–11, https://doi.org/10.1016/j.jbusres.2021.08.011.

Barnes, D. The Great Stink of Paris and the Nineteenth-Century Struggle Against Filth and Germs. Johns Hopkins University Press, 2006

Belich, James. "The Black Death and the Spread of Europe." In James Belich, and others (eds), *The Prospect of Global History.* Oxford: Oxford Academic, March 24,. 2016, online edn. https://doi.org/10.1093/acprof:oso/9780198732259.003.0006. Accessed Summer 2024.

Bolton, Jim L. "The World Upside Down: Plague as an Agent of Economic and Social Change." In W. M. Ormrod and Phillip Lindley (eds), *The Black Death in England,* edited by W. M. Ormrod and Phillip Lindley. Stamford: Paul Watkins, 1996.

Cohn, Samuel Kline. *The Black Death Transformed: Disease and Culture in Early Renaissance Europe*. London: Hodder Education, 2003.

Dai, Z. "Telehealth in Long-term Care Facilities During the Covid-19 Pandemic – Lessons Learned from Patients, Physicians, Nurses and Healthcare Workers." *BMC Digit Health* 1, no. 2 (2023). https://doi.org/10.1186/s44247-022-00003-y.

Erwan Messager, et al. "Two Millennia of Complexity and Variability in a Perialpine Socioecological System (Savoie, France): The Contribution of Palynology and SedaDNA Analysis." *Frontiers in Ecology and Evolution* 10 (16 Jun. 2022). https://doi.org/10.3389/fevo.2022.866781. Accessed December 1, 2023.

Gottfried, Robert S. *The Black Death: Natural and Human Disaster in Medieval Europe*. New York: The Free Press, 1983, 83–4.

Gunasekeran, Dinesh V., et al. "Digital Health during COVID-19: Lessons from Operationalising New Models of Care in Ophthalmology." *The Lancet Digital Health* 3, no. 2 (Feb. 2021). https://doi.org/10.1016/s2589-7500(20)30287-9.

Halliday, S. *The Great Stink of London: Sir Joseph Bazalgette and the Cleansing of the Victorian Metropolis*. Stroud: Sutton Publishing, 2001.

Jordan, D. P. *Transforming Paris: The Life and Labors of Baron Haussmann*. New York: The Free Press, 1995.

Kherlakian, B.S. (2016). Haussmann's three pronged modernization of Paris. Retrieved from https://www.acdemia.edu/37515739/Rationalization_Expansion_Embellishment_Haussmann_s_Three_Prolonged_Modernization_of_Paris

Killingray, David. "A New 'Imperial Disease': The Influenza Pandemic of 1918–9 and its Impact on the British Empire." *Caribbean Quarterly* 49, no. 4 (Dec. 2003): 30–49. https://doi.org/10.1080/00086495.2003.11829645.

Matsumoto, Ryusuke et al. "Determining What Changed Japanese Suicide Mortality in 2020 Using Governmental Database." *Journal of Clinical Medicine* 10, no. 21 (November 7, 2021): 5199. https://doi.org/10.3390/jcm10215199.

McMichael, Anthony J. "Paleoclimate and Bubonic Plague: A Forewarning of Future Risk?" *BMC Biology* 8, no. 1 (August 27, 2010). https://doi.org/10.1186/1741-7007-8-108.

Piret, Jocelyne and Guy Boivin. "Pandemics throughout History." *Frontiers in Microbiology* 11, no. 1 (January 15, 2021). www.ncbi.nlm.nih.gov/pmc/articles/PMC7874133/; https://doi.org/10.3389/fmicb.2020.631736.

Plößl, F., & Just, T. (2022). Lessons from the cholera in Paris and Hamburg. In T. Just & F. Plößl (Eds.), European cities after COVID-19: Strategies for resilient cities and real estate, Springer, 2022, 49–54.

Routt, David. "The Economic Impact of the Black Death." *Eh.net*, 2004. eh.net/encyclopedia/the-economic-impact-of-the-black-death/.

Solomon, S., Greenberg, J., & Pyszczynski, T. (2003). Fear of death and human destructiveness. Psychoanalytic Review, *90(4)*, 457–474.

Solomon, S., Greenberg, J., & Pyszczynski, T. (2015). The Worm at the Core: On the Role of Death in Life. Random House.

Sowards, Will. "How Did the Spanish Flu Pandemic Change Health and Medicine?" *Passport Health*, August 9, 2018. www.passporthealthusa.com/2018/08/how-did-the-spanish-flu-pandemic-change-health-and-medicine/.

Sowards, Will. "How the 1918 Spanish Flu Pandemic Links to World War I." *Passport Health*, April 13, 2020. www.passporthealthusa.com/2020/04/1918-spanish-flu-links-to-world-war-i/.

Spernovasilis, Nikolaos, et al. "Emerging and Re-Emerging Infectious Diseases: Humankind's Companions and Competitors." *MDPI, Multidisciplinary Digital Publishing Institute*, January 4, 2022. www.mdpi.com/2076-2607/10/1/98.

Spinney, L. (2020, March 7). The world changed its approach to health after the 1918 flu. Will it after the COVID-19 outbreak? TIME Magazine

Tarr, J. A. "Water and Wastes: A Retrospective Assessment of Wastewater Technology in the United States, 1800–1932." *Technology and Culture 25(2),* (1984): 226.

Thalassinou, Eleni, et al. "Biological Warfare Plan in the 17th Century—the Siege of Candia, 1648–1669." *Emerging Infectious Diseases* 21, no. 12 (December 2015). https://doi.org/10.3201/eid2112.130822. Accessed November 15, 2020.

Thompson, James Westfall. "The Aftermath of the Black Death and the Aftermath of the Great War." *American Journal of Sociology* 26, no. 5 (March 1921): 565–572. https://doi.org/10.1086/213206.

Tomes, Nancy. "'Destroyer and Teacher': Managing the Masses during the 1918–1919 Influenza Pandemic." *Public Health Reports* 125, no. 3_suppl (April 2010): 48–62. https://doi.org/10.1177/00333549101250s308.

Wallace, Rob. "Medical Innovations: From the 1918 Pandemic to a Flu Vaccine: The National WWII Museum: New Orleans." The National WWII Museum | New Orleans, The National World War II Museum, April 12, 2020. www.nationalww2museum.org/war/articles/medical-innovations-1918-flu.

Zentner, McLaurine H. "The Black Death and Its Impact on the Church and Popular Religion." *Academia*, 2015. www.academia.edu/31887760/The_Black_Death_and_Its_Impact_on_the_Church_and_Popular_Religion.

6

Slovenian Crime Fiction in the Time of the Covid-19 Pandemic and Neoliberalism

A Case Study of Imaginary Immunities

Primož Mlačnik

In this text, I present and analyze a Slovenian crime novel, *The Virus (Virus,* 2020*)*, written by Tadej Golob and chronologically placed in the period of the first wave of the Covid-19 pandemic. First, I present Slovenian crime fiction's history, its recent efflorescence represented by the most famous crime writer, Golob, and the social context of lockdown and right-wing political ascendancy. Second, I explicate the use of the immunitarian paradigm in the context of neoliberal pandemics, generally defined as the initial contradictory, self-destructive, individualized, and anti-communal (non)responses to the spreading of Covid-19. I also present the immunitarian tendencies of the detective genre at the level of the autoimmunizing detective narrative and the detective triad. Third, I present *The Virus* as a neoliberal crime novel with desocialized representations of crime, a socially immune neoliberal detective, and a fetishized detection process. Using John Cawelti's dichotomy between classic and hard-boiled detective stories, I delineate the ideological traits of a neoliberal detective. Although becoming individually immune to Covid-19 is discursively linked with immunity to social evil, the (pandemic) neoliberal detective paradoxically contributes to the public good by pursuing private interests. I show that the detection process in *The Virus* is fetishized, rendering the individualized and immune character of the detective redundant. Historically, this is a peculiar trait of Slovenian crime fiction, which needs some context.

The Revival of Slovenian Crime Fiction Amid the Covid-19 Pandemic and Rising Authoritarianism

In the second half of the nineteenth century and the first half of the twentieth century, only a handful of parodically distant crime novels and stories were published in the primarily rural Slovenian society. Slovenian crime fiction began its ascendancy in the 1980s and 1990s after the breakup of Yugoslavia and under the strong influence of postmodernism, which rendered the previously considered trivial genre closer to high literature than to popular fiction. Although crime novels of the late 1990s and early 2000s were preoccupied with questions of national identity, similarly to other European countries in transition and the thrall of globalism, parodically distant and experimentally metafictitious historical tradition prevented mass readership and lasting acclaim of Slovenian crime fiction until the second decade of the twenty-first century when a serial detective or crime novels have begun flourishing under the influence of widespread and well-read Scandinavian noir.

Tadej Golob, an ex-journalist who wrote for Playboy and an avid climber, resembling the Norwegian crime writer Jo Nesbo, finds himself in the eye of the efflorescent Slovenian crime fiction tornado. His first crime novel, *The Lake* (*Jezero*, 2016), was nominated for the Kresnik Award, annually bestowed for the best Slovene novel. Golob's crime series, featuring an incomprehensibly gloomy detective protagonist, Taras Birsa, an oxymoronic depiction of a Slovenian man or a mountaineer who is allergic to alcohol, is the most famous author, residing at the top of the Slovenian annual library loans and bookshop sales. Besides The Lake, which was adapted into a TV series in 2019 (designated as "subalpine noir" at The Sarajevo Film Festival), he wrote the novels *Lenin Park* (*Leninov park*, 2018), *The Valley of Roses* (*Rožna dolina*, 2019), and *The Virus*. Writing and reading a contemporary detective or crime novel against the backdrop of pandemics is generally rare. In Slovenia, *The Virus* presents a unique and precedential historical case. Golob, a pigeon in English, has managed to fly over the nest of the global neoliberal pandemics and the local ascent of authoritarian politics.

In Slovenia, the rapid spreading of Covid-19 and the consequential first social lockdown in March 2020 was accompanied by the ascendancy of a new (and old) authoritarian right-wing government led by Janez Janša's SDS (Slovenian Democratic Party). Janša was confirmed as the new prime minister by the

National Assembly on March 13th. On March 4th, the first case of the virus was confirmed, and as of March 30th, all public gatherings were banned, and movement was restricted to the municipality of residence. Slovenians have taken these measures with ambivalence. On the one hand, the extreme severity of the Covid-19 pandemic was on full display in the neighboring country of Italy, and anti-Covid-19 measures such as social distancing and other precautionary measures such as disinfection and the use of medicinal face masks were followed religiously. On the other hand, there were justified anxieties and later confirmed suspicions that the problematic Slovenian government would use the epidemics to spread their political power and strengthen the neoliberal state: "In the wake of the COVID-19 pandemic, public health and common welfare have become a matter of culture wars, and the fragmentation of the public sphere has made it increasingly difficult to conduct a rational political debate."[1]

From the perspective of the immunitarian modern paradigm, presented in the continuation, the Covid-19 pandemic is only another yet the most severe medicinal and immunological threat to the immunity of the Slovenian (also European and global) community. From the year 2015 onwards, such a threat was represented mainly by the image of an Other or a refugee, who was coming from the Middle East to threaten the Slovenian way of life, and often, indeed, discursively yet unjustifiably linked with diseases and as being exempted from legal and Christian laws. Therefore, it is somewhat symptomatic that the infectious appeal of this Slovenian police procedural matches not only with the spread of a contagious disease, which presents the threat to social and biological impurity, but also the return of the authoritarian right-wing social conservatism, which often uses the fascist semiotics of social purification.

The Modern Immunitary Paradigm and Neoliberalism in the Era of Pandemics

Although one must have reservations against biological metaphors of social phenomena because of the history of social Darwinism and the close relation of biological metaphors to the justification of racism and social inequality, I dare to make use of Derrida's distinction between immunity and autoimmunity, precisely because Derrida's dichotomy crosses with the idea of "the survival of the fittest," which is present in the discourses of authoritarian neoliberalism and the discourses of the Covid-19 pandemic.

Derrida wrote of an immunitary reaction as the production of antibodies against the foreign antigens that protect the immune system from destruction.[2] However, autoimmunity is a more interesting and contradictory case of protecting the immune system against its self-protection. Derrida defined the autoimmunitary process as "that strange behaviour where a living being, in quasi-suicidal fashion, itself works to destroy its own protection, to immunize itself against its 'own' immunity."[3] He linked autoimmunitary processes with the events following the September 11 terrorist attacks in 2001, and the reactionary American military intervention in the Middle East that ended up reproducing and regenerating terrorism, "the very thing it seek([ed]) to disarm."[4]

It is essential to know that immunization and autoimmunization can sometimes be intertwined. In trying to reach immunity, societies attempt to secure the sacred elements. However, by doing so, they can destroy their mechanisms of protection: "The indemnification of the unscathed is the price of immunity [. . .], and violence of sacrifice in the name of non-violence."[5] I argue that this intertwinement was at work in the pandemic crisis. The sacred of neoliberalism is the free market, and while the social, cultural, and educational institutions were closed, the production and consumption of material goods continued during the pandemic lockdown. However, because the "pandemic socialism" was still unimaginable, and workers continued to work in hazardous environments, it was hard to stop spreading the virus. In contrast, the neoliberal pandemic has only deepened the global socioeconomic crisis, raising unemployment and "aggravating the pre-existing inequalities."[6]

Esposito states that immunity is a medical, legal, social, political, and cultural category. At the same time, immunization (together with individualization and rationalization) can be thought of as a paradigm of modernity or as complex progressive processes of exemption of individuals and groups of individuals from the obligations of the community (taxes, laws, service, charges, etc.).[7] Being immune means being isolated and protected, "free of debt that binds [modern individuals] together."[8] While not directly addressing the category of autoimmunity, Esposito comes to the same conclusion as Derrida—immunity (*immunitas*) stands in direct opposition to the community (*communitas*): "Life is sacrificed to the preservation of life. In this convergence of the preservation of life and its capacity to be sacrificed, modern immunization reaches the height of its own destructive power."[9]

Šumonja argues that the pandemic itself should be considered a crisis of neoliberalism (or a neoliberal pandemic) for different interrelated reasons that have caused the pandemic. Firstly, the coronavirus itself was a product of "agroindustry's devastating impact on natural ecosystems,"[10] and globalization was a critical factor in the rapid spreading of the virus. Secondly, the neoliberal measures that have privatized and depleted the national healthcare systems worldwide in the last thirty years have vastly contributed to the health crisis. Thirdly, the initial so-called "epidemiological neoliberalism"[11] was crucial in the pandemic crisis. In other words, when the deadly virus started spreading, the neoliberal governments reacted in the worst possible way, pretending to "do nothing while making sure that the 'natural laws' of markets [kept] functioning, even if it mean[t] allowing people to get sick and die from 'just another flu.'"[12]

Thus, it can be argued that from the community's perspective, epidemiological neoliberalism is an autoimmunitarian process aimed at immunization of society by granting immunity to the free market and deepening the pandemic crisis. In contrast, the "crisis socialism" (government subsidies for wages, exemption from work, vaccination) benefits society's immunization. In contrast, both processes are part of the same coin—the Western neoliberal societies are returning to their "normal," dysfunctional biologically immune state yet within broken and depleted communities.

In the context of the immunitarian paradigm, crime fiction has a contradictory character regarding detective stories. It is structurally based on a linear narrative triangle of disturbance of social order, identification of the unlawful, and re-establishing the status quo of social order. In the classic detective story, an immune society is crimeless, and the detective is an immunologist who eliminates harmful "antigens." However, society is an abstract entity. Only murder in a small community establishes this community through collective and unidentified guilt. In this sense, the detective's role is autoimmunitary. His resolution of the detective case and murder mystery disperses the established community of individuals who start leading private lives once again. It subdues them to the workings of society, which will eventually lead to future crime. The latter is realized in the hard-boiled detective story, where the detective can never reach social immunity because crime is socially immanent, also permeating the immune and autoimmune detective character.[13]

Therefore, it is vital to place *The Virus* in the historical and theoretical context of neoliberal noir, which corresponds to the logic of pandemic neoliberalism because the solution of the detective case by the autoimmune detective is linked with (un)resolved pandemic crisis.

The Virus as a Neoliberal Crime Novel

Neoliberal noir presents "an active and negative response to neoliberalism [challenging] its commodified rhetoric of self-reinvention, self-investment, and self-maintenance."[14] Neoliberal noir "reveals creeping anxieties about the privatised risk,"[15] and portrays a non-signifying "affective atmosphere of capitalism,"[16] which permeates the plot, individual narratives and characters—all marked by a surplus of negative affects of everyday activities guided by cruelly optimistic fantasies about a good life.[17] However, *The Virus* does not challenge the contradictions of neoliberalism but awkwardly affirms them.

The plot consists of two overlapping and discontinuous narratives: the narrative of crime, its investigation and resolution, and the narrative of the detective's private life's ups and downs in his working and domestic environment, entrenched between the spread of Covid-19 and social lockdown. The first narrative revolves around the investigation of three sequential murders of men found in different regions of the Slovene countryside by the main detective character, Taras Birsa, and his colleagues from the Department for Bloody and sexual delicts, located in the capital, Ljubljana. The first victim is Stanislav Kovač, a widower, a retired civil engineer and an ex-patriarch of a broken family. His ex-wife committed suicide, his 25-year-old daughter Sabina Kovač is mentally ill and institutionalized, and his 23-year-old son Andrej Kovač is in prison for theft and drug trafficking. The second victim is Franko Tepina, a single vulcanizer. The third victim is a priest, Mirko Lamut. The homemade wine *cvíček*,[18] which keeps Stanislav's carcass afloat in his wine cellar, the first crime scene, presents the most important clue, deciphered by Taras's team. Once they investigate the troubled personal past of Stanislav, they realize that besides a tooth for Stanislav's bottles of red wine found at all three crime scenes, these men also share an affinity for rape. Using forensic help, Taras's incomprehensible genius and the interrogation of Sabina, Andrej, and other extended family members, Taras's team manages to reconstruct the murder mystery. The murderer is Andrej. By killing three men that were a part of his father's drunken rape circle in the past, he avenges the destiny of his sister.

The second narrative presents the seemingly perfect affluent life of Taras Birsa and his wife Alenka, a pediatrician co-owning a health clinic. Their lives are disturbed when they contract and spread the virus in their working communities by disregarding the safety precautions. Taras is almost responsible for the death of his colleague Brajc, who developed a severe illness after contracting the virus. Taras also runs into trouble at the police department, transformed by new politically recruited personnel, because he is documented cycling or violating the obligatory 14-day quarantine. Alenka would have lost her job and clinic ownership without Taras's violent intervention. However, the equilibrium of their private family life is not established with the resolution of the detective case, the end of the first wave of pandemics, or the end of the state's social lockdown. The resolution of problems inherent to the two narratives is not connected, and the gap between the private and public remains open. The detective Taras Birsa overcomes all trouble with dry wit, dour countenance, and fists like the dirty inspector Harry Callahan.

As the social lockdown has forcefully turned people into "stay-at-home" persons, *The Virus* reflects the general atmosphere of the Slovenian lockdown and indirectly addresses social and political events. *The Virus* itself is quite a "stay-at-home" and immunitary novel, linked with the immunitarian paradigm by the notion of represented xenophobia and general narrow-mindedness but also incest and parricide, which are two of the most anti-social human acts, directly opposing the constitution of human civilization.[19]

The plot never crosses the Slovenian border, and the only foreigner in the novel is an Iranian refugee, presented as a lazy economic opportunist[20], coincidentally found near the first crime scene and beaten by two hillbillies on account of his race. The members of Taras's detective team act as unreliable anthropological informants or as tourist guides of exotic destinations, as is typical for detectives in the time of a globalized crime novel.[21] However, they do not guide the Slovenian readers through an exotic land but around Slovenia, presenting the cliches about its beauty, culinary specialties, and folklore amid three murders in different peripheral towns.

Interestingly, Golob, the writer or the writer's alter-ego namesake Golob, the forensic pathologist, compares the virus with social evil: "Isn't it after all that each criminal act is just following the fundamental matrix of the virus? Isn't every evil a consequence of previous evil and its infection?"[22] Ideologically or epistemologically speaking, this puts Golob between the fictional paradigm of "social organicist criminology" (society is like a biological organism, and crime spreads like a virus between biological entities) and the imaginary "pandemic crisis criminology" (in times of pandemic social crisis, crime spreads like a virus). However, Golob's analogy and both fictional analogies, imagined by the author of this text, are false. During social lockdowns and the spreading of

Covid-19 worldwide, crime rates (of murders and robberies per se) have fallen drastically if one does not consider crimes of the nation-states and corporations.

Crimes investigated in *The Virus* occur in the Slovenian countryside and are characterized by their paradoxical character. In contrast, the depiction of the character of crime seems simplistic, outdated, and individualized or desocialized, as being committed, on the one hand, by psychologically pathological individuals (the rape circle, organized by Stanislav Kovač), as postulated in positivist criminology, and on the other hand by an opportunistic individual (Andrej Kovač), who "has lost his way," as posited in classic criminology. Crime or the three murders are committed by Andrej Kovač, who murders every time he is on furlough.[23] He has everything to lose and decides to do so for personal and ethical reasons. Mirroring the detective Birsa, Andrej takes the law into his own hands and provides the social justice the system cannot provide. In a similar contradictory fashion, the criminal Kovač murders out of private interests to protect the public good (he gets rid of three unsanctioned sexual offenders), resembling the basic logic of the trembling hand of Adam Smith. The latter postulated that the rich work toward harmonious social relations and abolish poverty by pursuing their selfish interests in an unregulated market, guided by the invisible, equalizing, and distributive hand.[24]

In *The Virus*, crime ultimately leads back to the family, possibly the only non-commodified and essential communal social institution of neoliberal society, thus revealing anxieties about its corruption. Sabina Kovač becomes mentally ill because of continuous sexual abuse from her father and two other men, but the mental hospital does not cure her. Andrej Kovač is behind bars, yet the prison does not rehabilitate him; quite the contrary, it turns him into a serial killer who also commits parricide. It turns him into an ambiguous figure toward whom the reader feels empathy since the rapists deserve the punishment that other legal institutions could not provide. Intentionally or accidentally, Golob shows that two different disciplinary institutions, part of the modern biopolitical project, work toward greater dehumanization.

The Neoliberal Detective in a Viral Crisis

The plot of *The Virus* is set against the development of Covid-19 epidemics in Slovenia, which gradually slips into the story, and Birsa, the detective, also functions as a neoliberal autoimmunologist or a neoliberal epidemiologist. In the context of neoliberalism as a social ideology, which fosters the values of freedom, personal responsibility, and autonomy, producing self-disciplined, self-optimizing, and achievement-oriented individuals that are active, competitive, and flexible.[25] Birsa takes care of his body by cycling, running, and climbing. He represents at once a neoliberal subject whose body must be formed, used, and measured,[26] which is often communicated through "macho imagery"[27] and the cultural ideal of a Slovenian man who does not drink alcohol or smoke. Even though Birsa is allergic to alcohol, being somewhat of a pathological abstinent, he has the psychological structure of a junkie, unable to function without his thrilling fix. In the world of crime novels, Birsa resembles Nesbo's ex-junkie Macbeth. In contrast, in the world of the market economy, where a junkie and a yuppie are homomorphous,[28] he also represents a yuppie. However, Birsa's thrilling fix is sports.[29]

As is typical for a neoliberal individual, Birsa is predominantly a consumer, not a citizen. In the first chapter, he buys a new bicycle and a new car.[30] The omniscient narrator says that he and his wife Alenka can afford to eat at any restaurant and take a taxi anytime.[31] The narrator also says that they are planning a trip to the Italian Alps, where the Slovenian upper-middle-class citizens (many of them were doctors) symbolically consumed the coronavirus and brought it to Slovenia. The first chapter sets the tone of the physically active, economically preoccupied, and flexible individual who is interrupted and called up for work on a detective case when he is at the cinema with his wife—a murder interrupts the private comfort of a Slovenian detective, who leaves his wife at the cinema and visits the police station.

As a neoliberal epidemiologist and a Covid-19 skeptic, Birsa and his wife do not take the virus seriously and contract it first. His wife, an irresponsible doctor, does not wear a face mask in her office. At the same time, Birsa spreads the virus among his colleagues. Since health is such a vital neoliberal commodity that being immunologically vulnerable seems like an insult, Taras is in selfish denial, scornful of the virus after developing typical symptoms of Covid-19.[32]

Birsa experiences the fear of the virus as shameful to his freedom, and he puts himself and his private interests, which include working and doing sports, before the public good: "'I am afraid . . .' he pulled a face (. . .). So what? Fuck you, you should be ashamed!"[33] It is, therefore, not surprising and entirely in line with the neoliberal ethos that Birsa puts the responsibility of one's health into the hands of the individual, displaying "rigid and selfish individualism"[34] and attributing the responsibility for deprivation and impoverishment to the most afflicted members of society.[35] In this case, Birsa scolds the undisciplined and bohemian colleague Brajc: "About Brajc and his fear of death . . . Last year, he suffered from a warning stroke. Did he do anything not to suffer from another one? By himself? Nothing."[36] On the one hand, Birsa is legally and morally immune, as if these are the two preconditions to becoming physically immune to the coronavirus. He does not take anti-Covid-19 measures seriously, does not wear a mask, does not practice social distancing, and even rides his bicycle during the obligatory 14-day quarantine while getting through the infection: "He is not going to stay home, even if he drops dead."[37]

Birsa does not feel any guilt or fear, which are two basic emotions linked with the obligations and prohibitions of any community.[38] His wife Alenka is not much different, although she is a victim of an attempt at a sneaky take-over of her private pediatric clinic by the co-owner Peter Ogris, who shares with the news media that he told her she should have stayed home in self-isolation after returning from Italy. At the same time, she declined and answered: "Do you know how much I spent in the Dolomites? Who will bring that in?"[39]

On the other hand, the measures from Taras and Alenka are autoimmune and contradictory, following the neoliberal ethos: money comes before health, and private good comes before the public good. Because the coronavirus endangered their way of life, which is based on freedom, autonomy, and enjoyment in affluent life, they almost destroyed their working communities. Taras infects the whole detective team, with Brajc getting seriously ill and nearly dying. Taras feels no remorse when he finds out that Brajc is in intensive care.[40]

The detective is pandemically corrupted and convinced that people die of the coronavirus because of their lack of self-discipline, inactivity, and lack of care for the body machine. Death became central to crime fiction at the beginning of the twentieth century when death and dying started to recede into the private sphere and the public rituals of mourning declined; Birsa is radicalizing the privatization of death by attributing responsibility for a weak immune system to an individual, which is in line with the initial neoliberal treatment of the pandemics. The 14-day self-isolation also delays the work on the detective case, although it has to be noted that Birsa's ignorance does not have any severe consequences in this regard. Brajc survives, and even though Birsa becomes one of the "corona-fools" documented on Facebook, photographed on his bicycle during the obligatory period of self-isolation, his status as the head detective remains undisputed.

The supremacy of the private above the public is also displayed in Alenka's working environment. After Ogris attempts to pummel Alenka through the media and take over the private health clinic, she simulates getting beaten by Ogris[41] to manipulate Taras into settling the score.[42] Taras, exempted from the legal law as he is, then threatens and beats up Ogris. As an atypical, neoliberal, hard-boiled detective, he uses physical violence not to catch the murderer (e.g., to force a confession or surrender) for the public good but to confront a family foe who threatens its well-being by immoral but legal means. The pandemic neoliberal detective paradoxically contributes to the public good by pursuing private interests.

From the historical sociopolitical and economic perspective, Slovenia presents a case of a schizophrenic nation, so to speak, a nation with socialist roots (communal) and increasing neoliberal (immune) tendencies. One could argue that the majority of Slovenian detectives are also "schizophrenic" in terms of genre (e.g., commissioner Benjamin Perko from the crime novels (1991–2009) of Sergej Verč and Inspector Martin Vrenko from the crime novels (2007–20) of Avgust Demšar), Taras Birsa being no exception—schizophrenic in terms of the difference between a classic, deductive, aristocratic, bohemian and eccentric, ethically disinterested and distant detective, and a more modern, violent and dirty, working-class and ethically involved detective.[43] Taras is, in a way, a typical hard-boiled detective, temperamental, macho and occasionally violent with a sadistic impulse, a personification and abhorrence of the law. However, in *The Virus*, he is not ethically involved in his murder cases, although in other novels from Golob's detective series, he is often engaged as a murder suspect himself and as someone who is ethically conflicted.

Birsa is also, in a way, a classic detective who uses rational faculties to solve complex crimes and mystifying narratives. However, his reasoning is largely unexplained and unknown to the reader and his colleagues. Tina notices this:

> "She got used to the fact that he never showed his thoughts and intentions. From now and then, she thought whether that was a part of his method (. . .) did he intend to act like someone who knows more even though he did not?"[44] From the neoliberal perspective and as a neoliberal detective, Birsa only enacts a famous neoliberal formula, which encapsulates the schizophrenia or bipolarity of the detective: "Fake it until you make it."[45]

The Slovenian government, during the first and even more during the second national lockdown in 2021, has closed all educational facilities and other public and cultural institutions while leaving the private economy running freely, mostly avoiding "pandemic socialism" or economic compensation for the infected workers, and therefore perpetuating the spread of the coronavirus. Detective

Birsa is an ill yet immune individual. On the one hand, he thinks that death is necessary for the inactive and undisciplined. On the other hand, he is trying to beat it by staying (pro)active. So much of the novel's attention is devoted to Birsa's self-maintenance that it seems as if his profession as a detective is just a game—an indispensable evil in his life.

Case Closed: The Journey From Self-Care to Fetishized Immunity

Walter Benjamin once observed that "in times of terror, when everyone is something of a conspirator, everybody will be in the position of having to play detective."[46] This is also true in *The Virus*. There are neither clear suspects nor a red herring in the novel, which means that except for Birsa's detective team and family, everyone is a suspect of murder as much as everyone potentially has the coronavirus. *The Virus* could not be any closer to Christensen's suggestive reformulation of Benjamin's thought "that in times of precarity, everyone is placed in the position of having to play detective as the practice of self-care."[47] Moreover, murder can only be solved after the neoliberal detective becomes immune in the medicinal and legal sense or when he overcomes the coronavirus infection and the hardships he had to overcome because of his violent actions. The aforementioned "social organicist criminology" and "pandemic crisis criminology" join forces when the police recognize a criminal pattern and attempt to prevent further murders by restricting movement between municipalities.[48]

Returning to the schizophrenic character of the Slovenian neoliberal detective, we can also observe an exciting polarity regarding the process or character of detection concerning the dichotomy between the classic detective and the hard-boiled detective. Classic detectives like Sherlock Holmes deploy their mental genius to protect the public good from private desires. The hard-boiled detective is himself ethically entangled in this protection. In contrast, the neoliberal pandemic detective such as Birsa, contradictory as it seems, protects the public good by pursuing his private interests, mirroring the activity and motives of the murderer, Andrej.

In other words, the classic and hard-boiled detectives had the role of "social immunologists," which were indeed not without contradiction, as already mentioned. However, the neoliberal pandemic detective Birsa is autoimmunitary, almost destroying his detective team and the health of many others he is trying to protect. The neoliberal detective pursues private interests, which magically leads the narrative toward solving the detective case and the distribution of justice.

Like a hard-boiled detective, Birsa uses physical violence to achieve personal goals. Unlike a classic detective, he does not reconstruct the mystifying narrative at the end of the story. In the detection process, he continuously follows the detective clues, which experts scrutinize from different scientific fields of natural sciences (forensic pathology, molecular biology, and medicine), which help him catch the suspected murderer. Although the story revolves around disciplinary institutions (the prison, the hospital, and the asylum), which calls for a more Foucauldian reading of the origins of crime, Birsa only uses the help of natural sciences for detective reasoning that remains hidden and eventually redundant, never revealed to the reader. The paradox and the questionable, redundant role of the detective become apparent when Andrej Kovač, the murderer himself, pleads guilty and, instead of Birsa, reconstructs the missing links of the crime narrative.

Derrida argued that "it is (the) terrifying but fatal logic of autoimmunity of the unscathed that will always associate science and religion."[49] This ideological field of the immunitarian paradigm is apparent in *The Virus*, precisely in the detective work or the processes of detecting the overlapping crime and Covid-19. On the one hand, all evidence and detective clues are minutely deconstructed by different natural scientists, rendering Taras Birsa a redundant detective. On the other hand, despite the abundant scientific proof, the majority of characters follow a naive belief that the coronavirus should not be taken too seriously, displaying the classic formula of fetishist disavowal: "I know well that things are not as they appear, but I still act as if they were."

Although *The Virus* represents and critiques actual events (government corruption and politicized substitutions of police personnel), and the writer draws an analogy between the proliferation of crime and the spreading of the coronavirus infections, the crime investigated by detective Birsa is oddly desocialized, depoliticized, and privatized, originating in incest and rape, transpiring in three murders of sex offenders. Furthermore, the novel completely avoids class struggle. By its treatment of the character of crime and the criminal, it fails to address how epidemiological neoliberalism "sharpen([s]) the social inequality by separating the healthy/productive from the unhealthy/unproductive parts of population along ethnic, racial and cultural lines."[50]

Such essence of crime represents the neoliberal ethos, resembling the logic of the invisible hand, which also manifests itself in the neoliberal detective epidemiologist and the criminal. Paradoxically, the detective and the criminal protect the public good by pursuing their private interests. However, only the detective is rewarded or exempted from the law, despite his autoimmunitary, destructive actions. The discrepancy between private and public good is accentuated by privileging natural sciences in detecting crime while ignoring the scientific proof in detecting the coronavirus.

From the perspective of neoliberalism, which fosters individualism and freedom, and from the perspective of modern immunitarian processes, which progressively exempt individuals from communal laws and ties, this pattern is rather odd. Suppose we consider the detective triad in crime novels and detective stories as a field of contested social ideas and cultural representations. In that case, the ultimate role of the neoliberal detective in *The Virus* is to protect the patriarchal institution of marriage or the traditional nuclear family, as if the stable heterosexual monogamous partnership will make Slovenians and the Slovenian society immune to the manifestations of evil.

The analyzed novel is indeed ambiguous. While it seems to present a critique of pandemic neoliberalism and the Slovenian right-wing authoritarian government on the manifest level, it latently reproduces neoliberal ideology by affirmatively linking it to cultural conservatism.[51] In the one last reiteration of Benjamin's observation on detective fiction in times of crisis, one could say that in the time of pandemic neoliberalism, everyone, including the dirty detective, attempts to affirm an evasive immunity to guilt, fear, and the coronavirus by the practice of self-care. This is why in *The Virus*, solving the murder mystery is linked with solving the pandemic crisis and why the autoimmune neoliberal detective eventually proves to be redundant to the detective narrative and happily domesticated in his family. The story ends abruptly when the murder mystery is solved, but the neoliberal and pandemic crisis does not end.

Notes

1 Ksenija Vidmar Horvat, "Conspiracy Theories and the Crisis of the Public Sphere: COVID-19 in Slovenia," *Javnost* 28, no. 2: 232, https: //doi. org/10.1080/13183222.2021.1921522.

2 Jacques Derrida, *Acts of Religion* (New York; London: Routledge, 2002), 80.

3 Giovanna Borradori, *Dialogues with Jürgen Habermas and Jacques Derrida* (Chicago: University of Chicago Press, 2003), 94.

4 Borradori, *Dialogues with Jürgen Habermas*, 99.

5 Derrida, *Acts of Religion*, 88.

6 Miloš Šumonja, "Neoliberalism is Not Dead—On Political Implications of Covid-19," *Capital & Class* 45, no. 2 (2021): 220, https://doi.org/10.1177/0309816820982381.

7 Roberto Esposito, "The Twofold Face of Immunity," *Crisis & Critique* 7, no. 3 (2020): 74, https: //www. crisiscritique.org/storage/app/media/2020-11-24/roberto-esposito.pdf.

8 Roberto Esposito, *Communitas: The Origin and Destiny of Community*, translated by the Board of Trustees of the Leland Stanford Junior University (Stanford: Stanford University Press, 2009), 13.

9 Esposito, *Communitas*, 14.

10 Šumonja, "Neoliberalism is Not Dead," 217.

11 Šumonja, "Neoliberalism is Not Dead," 217.

12 Šumonja, "Neoliberalism is Not Dead," 218.

13 Žižek Slavoj and Močnik Rastko, "Spremna beseda [Foreword]," in *Memento umori*, ed. Slavoj Žižek and Rastko Močnik (Ljubljana: Državna založba Slovenije, 1982), 301–4.

14 Christopher Breu and Elizabeth A. Hatmaker, "Introduction: Dark Passages," in *Noir Affect*, ed. Christopher Breu and Elizabeth A. Hatmaker (New York: Fordham University Press, 2020), 6.

15 Matthew Christensen, "Managed Risk and the Lure of Transparency in Anglophone African Detective Noir," *Textual Practice* 29, no. 2 (2015): 321, https: //www. Tandfonline . com/ doi/ abs/ 10.1080/ 0950236X.2014.993522.

16 Andrew Pepper, "Capitalism as Affective Atmosphere: The Noir Worlds," in *Noir Affect*, ed. Christopher Breu and Elizabeth A. Hatmaker (New York: Fordham University Press, 2020), 242.

17 Pepper, "Capitalism as Affective Atmosphere," 245.

18 *Cvíček* is a light, acidic red wine from the lower Carniola region made of various grape varieties, including white and red grape species.

19 Sigmund Freud, *Totem and Taboo*, translated by James Strachey (London; New York: Routledge, 2001), 153.

20 Tadej Golob, *Virus* [*The Virus*] (Novo Mesto: Goga, 2020), 404.

21 Slavoj Žižek, "Parallax," *London Review of Books* 25, no. 22 (November 20, 2003), https://www.lrb.co.uk/the-paper/v25/n22/slavoj-zizek/parallax.

22 Golob, *Virus*, 223.

23 Golob, *Virus*, 481.

24 Adam Smith, *The Theory of Moral Sentiments* (Indianapolis: Liberty Fund, 1984), 184–5.

25 Patrick Schreiner, *Podreditev kot svoboda: Življenje v neoliberalizmu* [*Subordination as Freedom: Life in Neoliberalism*] (Ljubljana: Krtina, 2019), 21.
26 Schreiner, *Podreditev kot svoboda*, 59.
27 Renata Salecl, *A Passion for Ignorance: What We Choose Not to Know and Why* (Princeton; Oxford: Princeton University Press, 2020), 8.
28 Vito Flaker, "Heroin use in Slovenia: A Consequence or a Vehicle for Social Changes," *Eur Addict Res* 8 (2002): 175, https://www.jstor.org/stable/26790208.
29 Golob, *Virus*, 10.
30 Golob, *Virus*, 11.
31 Golob, *Virus*, 15.
32 Golob, *Virus*, 189–90.
33 Golob, *Virus*, 195.
34 Vidmar Horvat, "Conspiracy Theories," 232.
35 Schreiner, *Podreditev kot svoboda*, 30.
36 Golob, *Virus*, 194.
37 Golob, *Virus*, 234.
38 Esposito, *Communitas*, 20–61.
39 Golob, *Virus*, 231.
40 Golob, *Virus*, 235.
41 Golob, *Virus*, 343.
42 Golob, *Virus*, 353.
43 John Cawelti, *Adventure, Mystery and Romance: Formula Stories as Art and Popular Culture* (Chicago; London: The University of Chicago Press, 1977), 80–161.
44 Golob, *Virus*, 48.
45 Salecl, *A Passion for Ignorance*, 124.
46 Walter Benjamin, *The Selected Writings, Vol. 4, 1938–1940*, translated by Edmund Jephcott (Cambridge, MA: Harvard University Press, 2006), 21.
47 Christensen, "Managed Risk and the Lure of Transparency," 318.
48 Golob, *Virus*, 357.
49 Derrida, *Acts of Religion*, 80.
50 Šumonja, "Neoliberalism is Not Dead," 223.
51 See Melinda Cooper, *Family Values: Between Neoliberalism and the New Social Conservatism* (New York: Zone Books, 2017).

References

Benjamin, Walter. *The Selected Writings, Vol. 4, 1938–1940*. Translated by Edmund Jephcott. Cambridge, MA: Harvard University Press, 2006.

Borradori, Giovanna. *Dialogues with Jürgen Habermas and Jacques Derrida*. Chicago: University of Chicago Press, 2003.

Breu, Christopher and Elizabeth A. Hatmaker. "Introduction: Dark Passages." In *Noir Affect*, edited by Christopher Breu and Elizabeth A. Hatmaker, 1–28. New York: Fordham University Press, 2020.

Cawelti, John. *Adventure, Mystery and Romance: Formula Stories as Art and Popular Culture*. Chicago; London: The University of Chicago Press, 1977.

Christensen, Matthew. "Managed Risk and the Lure of Transparency in Anglophone African Detective Noir." *Textual Practice* 29, no. 2 (2015): 315–33. https: //www. Tandfonline.com/doi/abs/10.1080/0950236X.2014.993522.

Derrida, Jacques. *Acts of Religion*. New York; London: Routledge, 2002.

Esposito, Roberto. *Communitas: The Origin and Destiny of Community*. Translated by the Board of Trustees of the Leland Stanford Junior University. Stanford: Stanford University Press, 2009.

Esposito, Roberto. "The Twofold Face of Immunity." *Crisis & Critique* 7, no. 3 (2020): 73–9. https://www.crisiscritique.org/storage/app/media/2020-11-24/roberto -esposito.pdf.

Flaker, Vito. "Heroin Use in Slovenia: A Consequence or a Vehicle for Social Changes." *Eur Addict Res* 8 (2002): 170–6. ttps://www.jstor.org/stable/26790208.

Freud, Sigmund. *Totem and Taboo*. Translated by James Strachey. London; New York: Routledge, 2001.

Golob, Tadej. *Virus* [*The Virus*]. Nova Mesto: Goga, 2020.

Pepper, Andrew. "Capitalism as Affective Atmosphere: The Noir Worlds." In *Noir Affect*, edited by Christopher Breu and Elizabeth A. Hatmaker, 222–40. New York: Fordham University Press, 2020.

Salecl, Renata. *A Passion for Ignorance: What We Choose Not to Know and Why*. Princeton; Oxford: Princeton University Press, 2020.

Schreiner, Patrick. *Podreditev kot svoboda: Življenje v neoliberalizmu* [*Subordination as Freedom: Life in Neoliberalism*]. Ljubljana: Krtina, 2019.

Smith, Adam. *The Theory of Moral Sentiments*. Indianapolis: Liberty Fund, 1984.

Šumonja, Miloš. "Neoliberalism is Not Dead – On Political Implications of Covid-19." *Capital & Class* 45, no. 2 (2021): 215–27. https://doi.org/10.1177 /0309816820982381.

Vidmar Horvat, Ksenija. "Conspiracy Theories and the Crisis of the Public Sphere: COVID-19 in Slovenia." *Javnost* 28, no. 2 (2021): 219–35. https://doi.org/10.1080 /13183222.2021.1921522.

Žižek, Slavoj. "Parallax." *London Review of Books* 25, no. 22 (November 20, 2003). https://www.lrb.co.uk/the-paper/v25/n22/slavoj-zizek/parallax.

Žižek, Slavoj and Močnik Rastko. "Spremna beseda [Foreword]." In *Memento umori*, edited by Slavoj Žižek and Rastko Močnik, 295–349. Ljubljana: Državna založba Slovenije, 1982.

7

A Postscript in Verse

Seven Circles of Self

Hassan Mekouar

1: At the Center, the "I"

Ever since the famous formula
The *Cogito Ergo Sum*
The "I" in the *cogito* and the *sum*
Has stood secure
Like a watch tower
Guarding against confusion
Between self and not self
The ultimate shield against illusion
And dream
All the tricks human senses can play
All the hallucinations
Physical as well as metaphorical
Sapient beings may be subjected to . . .
For centuries
The one unshakable truth
Has been the persistence of the "I"
Descartes' *ergo*
That even if all knowledge
May prove but a kind of dream or illusion
There will always be an "I" who knows
An "I" who may be dreaming or confused
But an "I" that cannot be taken for a "not I" . . .

2: When the "I" is "You" (and "Us")

But wait!
So many of us
Refer to ourselves
As "you"
When we write
Or when we speak
For instance
When we say "you" to ourselves
To mean "I"
As in:
You should have said Yes
You should have said Yes, my God!
You'll regret it all your life . . .
Or
You should have said No
You should have said No, my friend!
You'll regret it all your life . . .
Like the "friend" which is the self
The "you" in this case is obviously an "I"
A rhetorical device
We often resort to it
To create a mental space
However small
Between us and our thoughts
Or our actions
Just as we often use "we" instead of "I"
—Exactly as I am doing at this moment—
To generalize
Reach beyond the individual "I"
Making whatever the "I" thinks
Or does
Partake of the broader "you" or "we . . ."
Now, it must follow
This "I" is slightly less secure
At its core
Than Descartes would have liked
When the self starts extending, stretching

There is no telling where it will go
And how far it will reach . . .

3: I Entertain Myself & Keep Myself (a Little) Company

Look
How many people you know
Do *not* speak to themselves
Some of the time or all of the time
Aloud or in the silence
Of their own secret self? . . .
All these folks
Sane or (slightly) insane
Use an "I" of course
To address a "you"
While no physical "you" is anywhere near
They speak aloud
(Or more often in silence)
As they would
To any "you"
Singular or plural
Using all the inflections
Human language can muster . . .
They may inform themselves of things
They already know
They may share stories with themselves
And anecdotes
See what I did yesterday! . . .
Or amuse themselves with jokes
Now look what X asked me to do the other day! . . .
They try and muster courage
To do or not to do
Something or another
They attempt to persuade (or dissuade)
A listener who is also the speaker
Lining up all kinds or arguments
As in a court of law
Sometime they speak to themselves
To congratulate themselves

Other times it is blame they hurl
At the other "I" they don't like
You cruel creature! Why did you do that? Why? Why? . . .
Infinities of examples I can dream up
That all have in common
Situations in which
An "I" communicates with a "you"
Who is the same as the "I" speaking
A "you" who is the same as the "I"
Or is he
Is she? . . .

4: When the Gap Grows . . .

For too long
In our human history
And even after terms
Such as split personality
Or schizophrenia
Became common currency
Folks believed
—And in many places still believe—
A self may be possessed
Occupied by another
Or more
Different selves
Who for reasons beyond understanding
Decide to dwell
To live in another self . . .
The dweller-occupier
Is generally evil
Or at the least
Bothersome enough to cause
Periodic problems
To the self that is occupied
And to their kinfolks . . .
Different cultures have different concepts
Different names
For the occurrence
The "devil" and all his evil avatars

Being
The single universal symbol . . .
One good, god-fearing self
Is forced to cohabitate
With another evil self
Who may whisper suggestions
Instigate unspeakable actions
By the (supposedly) sane
Unwilling host self . . .
The devil did it
The devil did it . . .
This evil self must now be purged
At all costs
Exorcize, Exorcize
Destroy the body
To rid the soul of its evil occupant . . .
In our own cultural sphere
The concept of *Djinns*
Immediately comes to mind . . .
Miskīn or Miskīna
Is
Miskūn or Miskūna . . .
The poor one is "inhabited"
We know how these creatures
Who "live" in
Or within a human being
Possess separate identities
With names and such
And moods
Likes and dislikes
Moments when they show up
And moments when they hide
They sometimes even speak in accents
Or even in a language
The self itself cannot speak!
Oh how difficult it is to rid the self
Of such a cumbrous
—We may call it—
Alter self

Who drains the first self
Of all its resources . . .
And it is not rare
That the *djinn* or its female equivalent
The usually
Deceptively lovely *djinniya*
Is of the opposite gender
Which makes it so
That we now
Have two or more really separate selves
Dwelling in one
Selves as distinct
As two genders can be
LGBT notwithstanding . . .
So, when the gap grows
It follows
These sundry manifestations
Of the same self may express
Different personalities
While they belong each
To a different universe . . .
Now, will the real "I" please stand up?

5: Will the Real "I" Please Stand Up!

In the field that is ours
The boundless domain of literature
The writers we are taught are the greatest
The writers that we teach are the greatest
Are those where little or no trace of the self
Can be found in what they write
Where are you William Shakespeare?
In the characters you create
I am sure some part of your self
Lies somewhere
In one or more
Of your immortal creations
Male or female
But surely
If we were to ask any scholar

Which of the characters in all of Shakespeare
Is closest to the man Shakespeare
There would be
As many answers
As there are scholars of the poet
And scholars of his poems . . .
Even scholars of his sonnets
Disagree on the self in the sonnets
The speaker there
The "I"
Addressing that epicene "you."
And if in theory at least
Scholarship may be able
To identify the "you"
Based on internal and external evidence
I'm not sure it is capable
Of pinning down the real "I"
The speaker in each of the poems
The voice we call the persona
First, because the persona
Is not the poet
—We all know that—
The persona is a facet of the poet
But it is not the poet
Despite the artistry
To persuade
Or to sway
Whoever happens to be
That particular "you" . . .
Now
In order to create a persona
The poet must be able to experience
The feelings and moods of the persona
In order to convey
This or that emotion the persona may feel
The poet must become the persona
For at the very least
Part of the time
During the creative process

Or else it is the very self of the poetic persona
Which becomes
The true self
Of the creator of the persona.
Whichever way we look at it
The self
Assumed in the voice of a persona
Can never be entirely identical
To the self of the poet . . .

6: The Infinite Faces of the (Poetic) Self

When the poet writes
I sing myself and celebrate myself
In the classic entitled
"Song of Myself"
Even if he gives this self "singing" for us
The kind of ID
One might require for a passport say
A name
Walt Whitman
An age
I, now thirty-seven years old
An ethnic origin
Born here of parents born here the same
Physical traits
And details of his health
My respiration and inspiration, the beating of my heart, the passing of blood and air through my lungs
And so much more
Throughout the 52 sections
And all across the successive revisions
Of his *Leaves of Grass*
Even so
And from the start
Whitman states that *my* self is *your* self
For every atom belonging to me as good belongs to you
Because for him
Both the "I" and the "you"
Partake of this bigger self

A self that is
—To use the transcendental term
In fashion at the time—
"Divine" . . .
From this central poetic self then
The self of one Walt Whitman
Profession: poet
There emerge many selves
Not only the various personae
In his countless kaleidoscopic lists
Of men and women of all ages
And all walks of life
And death
That all are made to be part of the self
But also what we readers may call
The principal persona
The ubiquitous "I"
Who speaks the very first word in the poem.
This "I" also changes
If ever so slightly
From revision to revision of the poem
From Fifty-five to Eighty-one
Of that nineteenth century
The way any "I" evolves with time
And more . . .
Here then we can see a self
Roam and ramble and wander
In the dimensions of space
And society
And also in the dimension of time
A self re-created
Ad infinitum
Always one
And always much more than one . . .
When a self embraces so many selves
When the singular is so plural
Is so much more
Than a single monolithic "I"
Now, whenever the self thinks "I"

Speaks with the voice of a persona
That self becomes another . . .
Who is the real self then that uses the "I"?

7: The Problem with the Poet (According to Plato)

Perhaps we can now understand
Plato's problem with the poet
Why he thought the poet should be banished
From his well-ordered Republic
He believed
That real poetry
Compared to simple skill or talent
Or mere oratory
Requires some form
Of divine inspiration
And divine inspiration for him
Is a form of madness
Possession if you wish
No different a state from the temporary
Or permanent occupation of a self
By some other self
No different
From all the wanderings
And meanderings of the poetic self
I mentioned before . . .
When he composes true poetry
The poet is not himself
The poet is under an influence
Something much stronger is at work.
The poet has a vision
For reasons and at times
The poet cannot control
And the poet must give birth to that vision
Hence
The voice that an audience hears or reads
Does not belong entirely to the poet
A poem is the medium and the expression
Of more
Than a single, monolithic, Cartesian self . . .

Here we can perhaps attempt to sum up
This rambling reflection on the self
By one obsessed
With the elastic nature of self
Sum up perhaps
By stretching ever so little
René Descartes' formula
To something like this:
I think, therefore I am
I think, therefore you are
I think, therefore we are
You think, therefore I am
You think, therefore we are
Et cetera, et cetera . . .

Harhoura, September 2015

Index

About the Editors

Mohamed Belamghari is a Moroccan associate professor of English language and literature at the faculty of Letters and Humanities of Ibn Zohr University in Morocco. His fields of academic interest are cultural and literary studies, Moroccan literature, culture & civilization, and colonial and postcolonial studies, among others.

Bouchra Benlemlih is Professor of English and postcolonial studies at the Faculty of Letters and Humanities, Ibn Zohr University, Agadir, Morocco, where she is coordinator of the research group on Ethics, Representation, and Politics in Literature and Culture (EREPLIC). Her present research interests include comparative literature, postcolonial studies, cultural studies, North African studies, American studies, and globalization. She has supervised PhD research on these fields of study. Benlemlih is the author of *Paul Bowles's Literary Engagement with Morocco: Poetic Space, Liminality, and In-Betweenness* (2018). She is also the editor of *Global Identities in Transit: The Ethics and Politics of Representation in World Literatures and Cultures* (2022).

Mustapha Kharoua is Associate Professor of literature and cultural theory at the Faculty of Languages, Arts and Humanities, Ibn Zohr University. His thesis *Traumatic Realism in Diasporic African Writing* was published by the University of Eastern Finland in 2016. His research interests are in the areas of postcolonial trauma studies, post-Andalusian criticism and migration studies. Some of his published articles include "Traumatic Realism and the Retrieval of Historical Value in Chimamanda Ngozi Adichie's Half of a Yellow Sun" (2015), "Abdulrazak Gurnah's By the Sea: Unbelonging and the Trauma of Imprisonment" (2016). "Postcolonial Writings on African Diaspora: On Collective Recovery" (2018), "'Epistemicide' and 'Memoricide', Legalized Destruction in the Arab/Muslim World" (2023), and "Rerouting Postcolonial Studies: A Post-Andalusian Critique of Western Modernity" (2023). He has served as a reviewer with the *Digest Journal of Middle Eastern Studies*. He has also been a member of the editorial board of the volume *Identities in Transit: Ethics and Politics of Representation in World Literatures and Cultures* published in collaboration with Lexington Books in 2022.

About the Contributors

Moulay Abdessadek Ahlbentaleb is a Moroccan researcher with over twenty-six years of teaching experience, currently serving as Associate Research Professor at FLASH, Ibn Zohr University in Southern Morocco. He is currently engaged in postdoctoral research at Utrecht University, focusing on early forms of inclusivity of Moor alterity on the English Renaissance stage. His research interests also include Jewish studies, criticism of Western paradigms of thought, and the Islamization of knowledge. Ahlbentaleb has published several articles in Arabic and English and recently co-edited a book on self-writing in postcolonial criticism.

Rachid Benharrousse is Research Fellow at the School of Global Affairs and Public Policy at the American University in Cairo. He has a PhD in migration studies from Mohammed V University in Rabat. His research focuses on migration, neoliberalism, necropolitics, and infrastructure. His international experience includes roles such as Don Lavoie Fellow at the Mercatus Center, George Mason University, and Research Director at Palah Light Lab, The New School. Benharrousse has also held positions as a Research Fellow at the African Academy for Migration Research (AAMR), University of Witwatersrand, and as a researcher at the Berkman Klein Center for Internet & Society, Harvard University & Digital Asia Hub. Benharrousse's early career was marked by his role as an Early Career Researcher with the Association of Middle Eastern Women's Studies (AMEWS) and as a Graduate Researcher at the Paris Institute for Critical Thinking. He also contributed as a lab researcher at Palah Light Lab & Amatryx Lab, University at Buffalo, SUNY.

Agostino Cera is Associate Professor of theoretical philosophy philosophy in the Dipartimento di Studi Umanistici at the Università di Ferrara. His research focuses on German thought between the nineteenth and twentieth centuries (Löwith, Heidegger, Anders, Nietzsche), philosophical anthropology, philosophy of technology, philosophy of cinema, and, more recently, the Anthropocene. His most recent books are *Nella società pandemica. Prove tecniche di tecnocosmo* (2022) and *A Philosophical Journey into the Anthropocene: Discovering Terra Incognita* (2023). Further information here: https://ferrara.academia.edu/AgostinoCera

Sidi Mohamed El Hassani is a qualified academic specializing in sociology and currently serves as a full-time lecturer in the Department of Sociology at the Faculty of Letters and Human Sciences, Sais, affiliated with Sidi Mohamed Ben Abdellah University in Fez. Dr. El Hassani holds a PhD in sociology sociology from Cadi Ayyad University in Marrakech. His academic qualifications further include a high diploma in urban planning from the National Institute of Urban Planning in Rabat, a master's degree in sociology of organizations organizations from the Faculty of Letters and Human Sciences in Marrakech, and a diploma in philosophy from the École Normale Supérieure in Meknes. His research interests encompass the sociology of organizations, social action, the anthropology of solidarity, and the study of social bonds. He has published numerous scholarly articles and studies in both Arabic and French in academic journals and edited volumes in the fields of sociology and anthropology.

Anouar Majid is Professor Emeritus of English at the University of New England. He is the author of many critically acclaimed academic books on the West and Islam. He has published major scholarly articles and has contributed opinion pieces to the Chronicle of Higher Education, the New York Times (with a colleague), and other national and international publications.

Hassan Mekouar is Professor Emeritus at Mohammed V Universit, Rabat, Morocco. He holds a licence degree in English and TEFL from Mohammed V University in Rabat (Faculty of Letters and ENS), a master's master's in English from Ohio University and a Brown University PhD. His academic career, from 1969 to 2011 combined teaching (American literature, literary criticism) and university administration (English Department chair, 1976 to 1981; dean of the Faculty of Letters in Rabat from 1982 to 1989 and rector at Mohammed I University in Oujda from 1989 to 1997. He published several collections of verse, all in English: The Future Remains, Parts I, II, and III (1999–2001), *The Wings of the Walrus* (2003), *Stories in (Very) Free Verse* and *7* (a twin collection, 2006), *Poems* 1969-2013 (2014) in 2 vols., and most recently, *Soft Sue & Other* (Goodbye) Poems (2021).

Primož Mlačnik, a pedagogue and researcher in cultural studies, is an assistant professor (docent) at the University of Nova Gorica. He earned his PhD from the University of Ljubljana, where he authored a scientific monograph, *Poročilo o melanholiji: primer Kafka* (2020). Currently, he is engaged in the research project *Shapes of Shame in Slovenian Literature* (2025–2028) and previously contributed to *Transformations of Intimacy in Slovenian Literary Discourse* (2021–2024). He has published in Slovenian scientific journals such as *Slavia Centralis, Jezik in slovstvo, Družboslovne razprave, Filozofski vestnik,* and *Studia Historica Slovenica,* as well as in international publications including *Caitele Echinox, Przekłady Literatur Słowiańskich, European Journal of Interdisciplinary Studies,* and *Communist and Postcommunist Studies.*

Sara Tabza is a Moroccan doctoral researcher in comparative literature studies at the Faculty of Letters and Humanities of Ibn Zohr University in Morocco. Her fields of academic interest are cultural and literary studies and comparativestudies in literature. She is as deeply engaged with existentialism and hermeneutics as she is with social psychology.

www.ingramcontent.com/pod-product-compliance
Ingram Content Group UK Ltd.
Pitfield, Milton Keynes, MK11 3LW, UK
UKHW020208290926
15470UKWH00001B/73

9 798216 380443